DYSPHAGIA
Assessment and Treatment Planning
WORKBOOK
A TEAM APPROACH

FIFTH EDITION

DYSPHAGIA
Assessment and Treatment Planning
WORKBOOK
A TEAM APPROACH

FIFTH EDITION

Julie Barkmeier-Kraemer, PhD, CCC-SLP
Rebecca Leonard, PhD, CCC-SLP

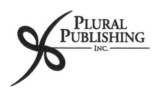

PLURAL
PUBLISHING
INC.

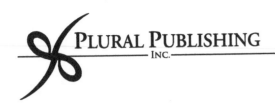

PLURAL PUBLISHING
INC.

9177 Aero Drive, Suite B
San Diego, CA 92123

email: information@pluralpublishing.com
website: https://www.pluralpublishing.com

Library of Congress Cataloging-in-Publication Data:
ISBN-13: 978-1-63550-496-5
ISBN-10: 1-63550-496-1

Contents

Contents

Introduction

After teaching Dysphagia for 14 years at the University of Arizona, I find that the common denominator across every semester save for my most recent one was a desire for a textbook and course format that integrated fundamental information about the anatomy and physiology of the aerodigestive tract into clinically relevant knowledge needed to problem-solve the diverse range of individuals with feeding and swallowing problems. After using several textbooks that did not fully meet my needs, I found the Leonard and Kendall textbook and discovered that it contains nearly every element needed for training speech-language pathologists in dysphagia. I implemented the second edition of the Leonard and Kendall textbook in my graduate course on Dysphagia and found the magical combination of basic fundamentals as well as evidence-based models of interdisciplinary clinical practice. The contributions from every professional on the University of California–Davis (UCD) Voice, Speech, and Swallowing team added the necessary contribution of information from professionals in otolaryngology, nursing, dietary, speech-language pathology, and gastroenterology. The textbook also integrates a synopsis of the most recent and relevant literature about deglutition to propose evidence-based methods of assessment and treatment approaches. This continuity of update and revision to incorporate the latest evidence-based approach and advancements in the science and technology of clinical services continues to be a unique contribution of the most recent fifth edition of the Leonard and Kendall textbook, *Dysphagia Assessment and Treatment Planning*.

This workbook was previously created to facilitate retention and improved implementation of content within the *Dysphagia Assessment and Treatment Planning* textbook. Based on feedback received by prior users of the workbook in academic classrooms, we have added course-friendly teaching and examination materials including online media for students and instructors on the PluralPlus companion website. Lecture materials are updated to incorporate revised materials in the textbook for inclusion in a Dysphagia course. The workbook mirrors the *Dysphagia Assessment and Treatment Planning* textbook's reorganization of chapters. The format of the workbook also maintained the prior student-friendly approach for facilitating the retention and application of information contained within the text. In addition, the workbook provides a separate updated set of quiz/exam questions and key responses for each textbook chapter for use by course instructors. The prior workbook material providing instruction on qualitative and quantitative approaches to analyzing videofluoroscopic studies are also updated and are available online including case-based examples.

We hope that the incorporation of online clinical and teaching materials for the textbook and workbook provides improved instructional course materials and clinically relevant approaches for learning assessment and treatment approaches to dysphagia.

JB-K

Acknowledgments

The authors gratefully acknowledge the contributions of colleagues at the UCD and at the University of Arizona who initially provided feedback on several of the original chapter materials developed for use in the workbook. We are also grateful to those providing feedback directly and indirectly regarding the use of the original workbook in an academic dysphagia course. Without this feedback, the ideas for the current range of course-based online materials would not have occurred. The co-editors of the textbook, Drs. Rebecca Leonard and Katherine Kendall, continue to be a source of inspiration by setting a standard for incorporating evidence-based practice and interdisciplinary expertise within their textbook including recruitment of new chapter authors with relevant content expertise. Their textbook offers one of the only such models of dysphagia practice that implements the recommended standard of care within a medical setting. We are honored to offer this supplementary set of learning materials to complement their superb model of dysphagia assessment and treatment. We would also like to acknowledge and thank our team of students and colleagues in the Voice, Airway, Swallowing Translational (VAST) Research Lab and Utah Voice Disorders Center who contributed importantly to the review, critique, and assistance toward completing this revised edition of the workbook. Specifically, we would like to thank and acknowledge the following contributors toward the revised workbook content and updated media and case examples: Kaitlyn Dwenger, Miranda Wright, Maya Stevens, Beth Lanza, Leann Smith, and Derrik Legler. Finally, thank you to all of the colleagues and students who have provided valuable comments and suggestions about their experience with the workbook materials for training and teaching purposes. We are hopeful this revised workbook and textbook bundle meets the needs and desires of all who have adopted them for learning, teaching, training, and reference purposes.

Multimedia List

1

Anatomy and Physiology of Deglutition Questions

1. Define the following terms.

   a. Deglutition

   _____

   _____

   b. Feeding

   _____

   _____

   c. Mastication

   _____

   _____

   d. Swallowing

   _____

   _____

   e. Bolus

   _____

   _____

   f. Aspiration

   _____

   _____

   g. Laryngeal penetration

   _____

   _____

   h. Residue

   _____

   _____

   i. Dysphagia

   _____

   _____

2. Match the following physiologic descriptions to their respective phase of deglutition.
   A. Preparatory
   B. Oral
   C. Pharyngeal
   D. Esophageal

   _____ Propulsion of the bolus into the pharynx

   _____ Mastication of the bolus

   _____ Transportation of the bolus through the esophagus to the stomach

   _____ The bolus is mixed with saliva

   _____ Transportation of the bolus through the pharynx into the esophagus

   _____ Airway closure occurs associated with cessation of respiration

   _____ The soft palate begins to elevate as the posterior tongue depresses

   _____ Bolus propulsion occurs through coordinated peristaltic contraction of both smooth and striated muscle

3. The skeletal framework that supports mastication includes all of the following bones EXCEPT the
   a. mandible.
   b. maxilla.
   c. palatine.
   d. frontal.

4. The bony nasal septum is formed by these bones (fill in the blanks).

   a. _____

   b. _____

5. Match the following phases of deglutition with the correct image in Figure 1–1.

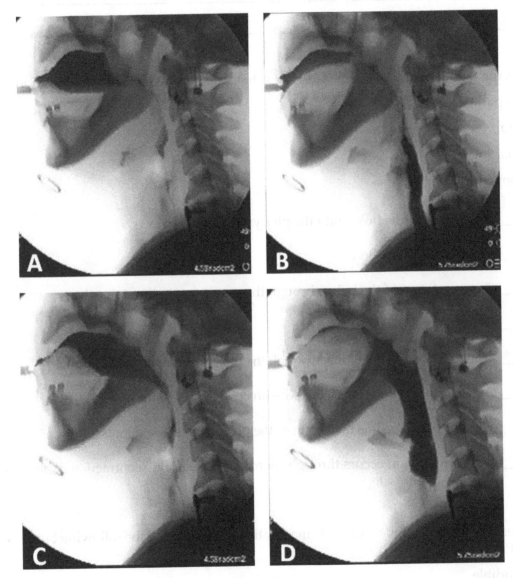

Figure 1–1

_____ Preparatory   _____ Pharyngeal

_____ Oral   _____ Esophageal

6. The floor of the nasal cavity is formed by these bones (select all that are correct).
   a. Ethmoid
   b. Nasal
   c. Palatine
   d. Maxilla

7. The middle and superior conchae provide the lateral nasal skeletal framework for the middle and superior turbinates that extend into the nasal cavity from this bone.
   a. Sphenoid
   b. Maxilla
   c. Ethmoid
   d. Palatine

8. Identify all of the skull bones comprising the cranium.

   _____

   _____

9. Identify the only mobile facial bone of the skull and the name of its joint.

   _____

   _____

10. Identify the cervical vertebrae typically associated with the location of the upper esophageal sphincter prior to onset of a swallow.

   _____

   _____

11. Identify all of the facial bones that form the skeletal framework for the oral cavity.

   _____

   _____

12. Identify the bone and particular portion of that bone through which the receptor organs for smell pass into the olfactory nerve.

_____

_____

13. Identify the muscles in Figure 1–2.

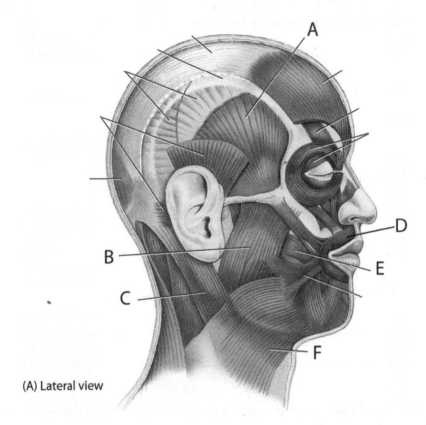

(A) Lateral view

Figure 1-2

A _____

B _____

C _____

D _____

E _____

F _____

14. Identify the structures in Figure 1–3.

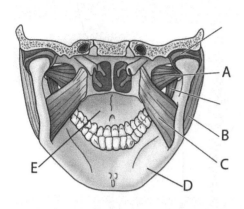

(D) Posterior view of viscerocranium

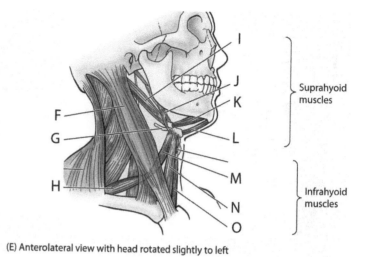

(E) Anterolateral view with head rotated slightly to left

Figure 1–3

A _____

B _____

C _____

D _____

E _____

F _____

G _____

H _____

I _____

J _____

K _____

L _____

M _____

N _____

O _____

15. Identify the structures in Figure 1–4.

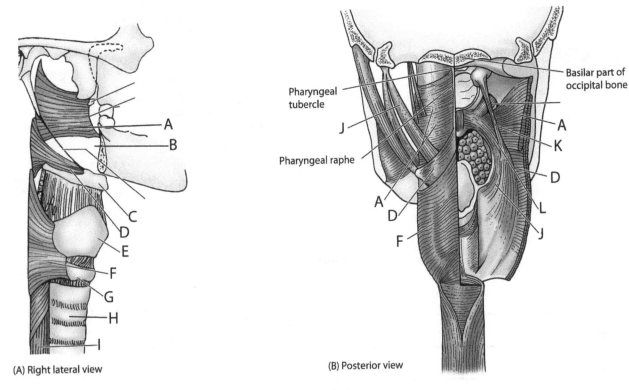

(A) Right lateral view

(B) Posterior view

Figure 1–4

A _____

B _____

C _____

D _____

E _____

F _____

G _____

H _____

I _____

J _____

K _____

L _____

16. Identify the muscle(s) that elevate(s) the mandible during mastication and the source of innervation for each.

    _____

    _____

    _____

17. Identify the muscle(s) that depress(es) the mandible during mastication and the source of innervation for each.

    _____

    _____

18. Identify the muscles within the anterior (a) and posterior (b) faucial pillars.

    a. _____

    b. _____

19. Identify all of the following facts that are characteristic of saliva.

    _____ Normal salivary secretion ranges from 1.0 to 1.5 L per day.

    _____ Saliva contains an enzyme for digesting starches.

    _____ Saliva only serves the purpose of lubrication of dry foods.

    _____ Saliva controls pathogenic bacteria responsible for dental caries.

    _____ Saliva is only produced by the parotid glands.

    _____ Saliva contains mucus for lubrication.

    _____ Innervation to salivary glands is supplied from sympathetic nervous system pathways.

20. Identify the muscle that elevates the soft palate and the source of its innervation.

    _____

    _____

21. Identify the muscles that contract to prevent forward pressure escape (i.e., out of the mouth) during the oral phases of deglutition and their source(s) of innervation.

_____

_____

22. Identify the three major muscles lining the posterior pharyngeal wall.

_____

_____

23. Identify the two portions of the inferior constrictor muscle of the pharynx and identify how their muscle function differs.

_____

_____

24. Identify all of the intrinsic tongue muscles and their source of innervation.

_____

_____

_____

25. This muscle elevates the pharynx during the pharyngeal swallow.

_____

_____

26. Identify the adductor muscles of the larynx.

_____

_____

27. Identify the abductor muscle(s) of the larynx.

_____

_____

28. Identify the three levels of folds in the larynx that close during the pharyngeal phase of deglutition.

_____

_____

29. Onset of swallowing begins with contraction of this muscle first.

_____

_____

30. Identify the group of muscles referred to as the "leading complex."

_____

_____

_____

31. Match the nerve providing motor innervation to each of the following muscles (each nerve may be correct for more than one muscle or may not be used at all).

A. CN V (trigeminal)

B. CN VII (facial)

C. CN IX (glossopharyngeal)

D. CN X (vagus), internal branch SLN

E. CN X (vagus), external branch SLN

F. CN X (vagus), RLN

G. CN X (vagus), pharyngeal plexus

H. CN X (vagus)

I. CN XII (hypoglossal)

J. Ansa cervicalis plexus (C1–C4)

_____ Levator veli palatini   _____ Palatopharyngeus

_____ Tensor veli palatini   _____ Anterior digastric

_____ Orbicularis oris   _____ Posterior digastric

_____ Buccinator   _____ Masseter

_____ Styloglossus   _____ Temporalis

_____ Superior constrictor   _____ Medial pterygoid

_____ Middle constrictor   _____ Lateral pterygoid

_____ Inferior constrictor   _____ Thyroarytenoid

_____ Mylohyoid   _____ Sternohyoid

_____ Stylohyoid   _____ Cricothyroid

_____ Geniohyoid   _____ Thyrohyoid

_____ Palatoglossus   _____ Posterior cricoarytenoid

32. Match the nerve providing sensory innervation for each structure or region in the following text (each nerve may be correct for more than one structure or region or may not be used at all).

A. CN I (olfactory)

B. CN V (trigeminal)

C. CN VII (facial)

D. CN IX (glossopharyngeal)

E. CN X (vagus), internal branch SLN

F. CN X (vagus), external branch SLN

G. CN X (vagus), RLN

_____ Taste to the anterior two-thirds of the tongue

_____ Taste to the posterior one-third of the tongue

_____ General sensation to the oral cavity

_____ General sensation to the faucial pillars

_____ General sensation to the face and lips

_____ General sensation to the oro- and laryngopharynx (a.k.a., hypopharynx)

_____ General sensation to the laryngeal vestibule and surface of the vocal folds

_____ General sensation to the subglottal portion of the vocal folds and trachea

_____ Sense of smell

33. Identify the portions of the cortex associated with speech movements and oral phases of swallowing.

_____

_____

34. Identify the subcortical sites associated with triggering or modifying swallowing.

_____

_____

_____

35. Identify all of the following characteristics that are true of the swallowing central pattern generator.

_____ Consists of a group of neurons within the reticular formation of the brainstem

_____ Receives afferent input from the trigeminal (V), glossopharyngeal (IX), and vagus (X) nerves

_____ Triggers a swallow pattern in response to stimulation of the superior laryngeal nerve branch of the vagus nerve (SLN)

_____ Triggers chewing with stimulation of the glossopharyngeal nerve

_____ Resides only within the pons portion of the brainstem

_____ Includes the nucleus tractus solitarius as the principal sensory nucleus involved in triggering the coordinated motor output

_____ Does not overlap with groups of neurons involved in respiration

_____ Includes coordination of a complex sequence of motor output from the hypoglossal (XII) nucleus and nucleus ambiguus (X) to produce the oropharyngeal swallow

_____ The dorsal swallowing group is composed of the motor nuclei of the nucleus ambiguus

_____ The ventral swallowing group receives sensory input that contributes to triggering the swallow

_____ Interneurons within the ventral swallowing group serve to distribute and coordinate activation of the motor neurons activated during swallowing

_____ Trigeminal and hypoglossal motor nuclei are only connected to interneurons within the ventral swallowing group

_____ Bilateral coordination of motoneuron pools is thought to occur via interneurons within the trigeminal and hypoglossal motor nuclei

36. A bolus is transported from the pharynx to the stomach via the _____.

37. These two components of the pharyngeal phase of swallowing are important for adequate opening of the upper esophageal sphincter so that the bolus can clear the pharynx into the esophagus.

_____

_____

_____

38. Identify the name of the two high-pressure segments located at the entry and exit from the esophagus.

_____

_____

39. Indicate whether the following statements are true or false (circle one) regarding the esophagus.

TRUE or FALSE: The adult human esophagus is 18 to 25 cm in length.

TRUE or FALSE: The esophagus connects the trachea to the stomach.

TRUE or FALSE: The esophagus remains flattened or collapsed between swallows.

TRUE or FALSE: The esophagus is a muscular tube with cervical, thoracic, and abdominal regions.

TRUE or FALSE: The muscularis propria portion of the esophagus is composed only of smooth muscle.

TRUE or FALSE: Esophageal peristaltic contraction is a volitional response.

TRUE or FALSE: Esophageal peristalsis can only be triggered by an oropharyngeal swallow.

TRUE or FALSE: Tertiary peristalsis can only occur in the smooth muscle portion of the esophagus and is unrelated to extrinsic innervation.

TRUE or FALSE: Contraction of esophageal striated muscle is innervated by the motor neurons within the nucleus ambiguus, whereas smooth muscle contraction is controlled autonomically.

TRUE or FALSE: Once the esophageal peristaltic wave is initiated, it is an all-or-none phenomenon that does not dissipate until it reaches the lower esophageal sphincter.

40. CLINICAL CHALLENGE QUESTION: Susan exhibits a gurgly voice quality after eating a meal, suggestive of bolus residue on the surface of her vocal folds. During a dynamic videofluoroscopic swallow study, Susan exhibits deep penetration of bolus materials to the level of the vocal folds without evidence of a respiratory protective response of coughing or throat clearance of the materials. As such, bolus residue is observed in the laryngeal vestibule after the swallow. Which sensory nerve appears impaired?

_____

_____

_____

_____

_____

41. CLINICAL CHALLENGE QUESTION: Stan has poorly controlled chronic obstructive pulmonary disease and has a history of frequent bouts of aspiration pneumonia. During your clinical evaluation at bedside, you notice that Stan is on oxygen and exhibits a rapid breathing rate. He complains of dyspnea, or air hunger, during tidal breathing that worsens upon physical exertion. Stan also complains that his dyspnea worsens during meals. Given Stan's history of frequent aspiration pneumonia, what reason might you consider as the primary cause?

_____

_____

_____

_____

_____

2

Head and Neck Physical Exam Questions

1. Identify all of the following patient complaints that are considered examples of dysphagia symptoms.

    _____ I cough and choke during meals.

    _____ I have been gaining too much weight.

    _____ I feel like there is something in my throat after I eat and I have to clear my throat to get it out.

    _____ My voice changes when I eat and I sound gurgly.

    _____ I get frequent migraine headaches.

    _____ I have severe allergies and postnasal drip.

    _____ My child refuses to eat and cries during meals.

    _____ Food sticks in my throat.

    _____ My vision has worsened during the past year.

    _____ I have a hard time understanding my spouse when he/she talks to me.

    _____ It hurts when I swallow.

    _____ It takes me about an hour to finish a meal because I need to take small bites and chew my food really well.

    _____ I only eat soup or drink protein drinks because meat and vegetables stick in my throat.

2. The head and neck physical examination by the physician is to determine changes in eating that may be explained by changes in

    a. _____

    b. _____

    c. _____

3. The three main components of the physician's examination include

    a. _____

    b. _____

    c. _____

4. Match the following symptoms to their most likely etiology.

   A. Antihistamines and antinausea medications

   B. Impaired vocal fold approximation or mobility

   C. Weak or impaired pharyngeal swallow; pharyngeal residue

   D. Gastroesophageal reflux

   E. Fibrosis and edema

   F. Aspiration

_____ Heartburn, indigestion, or feeling a lump in the throat

_____ Dry mouth (xerostomia)

_____ Reduced range of motion of the jaw after radiation therapy (trismus)

_____ Coughing and choking during meals

_____ Breathy voice quality, lose air quickly when talking

_____ Food sticks in my throat that needs to be cleared by drinking water

5. Parasympatholytic medications <u>INCREASE</u> or <u>REDUCE</u> (circle one) salivary production, resulting in <u>DROOLING</u> or <u>XEROSTOMIA</u> (circle one).

6. Parasympathomimetic medications <u>INCREASE</u> or <u>REDUCE</u> (circle one) salivary production, resulting in <u>DROOLING</u> or <u>XEROSTOMIA</u> (circle one).

7. Dopaminergic medications <u>INCREASE</u> or <u>REDUCE</u> (circle one) salivary production, resulting in <u>DROOLING</u> or <u>XEROSTOMIA</u> (circle one).

8. Tricyclic antidepressant medications <u>INCREASE</u> or <u>REDUCE</u> (circle one) salivary production, resulting in <u>DROOLING</u> or <u>XEROSTOMIA</u> (circle one).

9. <u>TRUE</u> or <u>FALSE</u> (circle one): Disturbances in glycemic control, such as occur in people with diabetes mellitus, can reduce salivary flow, resulting in oral dryness.

10. Identify side effects of a dry mouth (xerostomia).

_____

_____

_____

11. Select all of the following observations that are completed during examination of cranial nerves I–VII.

_____ Symmetry of the face

_____ Sensitivity of the tongue to touch

_____ Movement of the lips and eyelids

_____ Symmetry and tone of the tongue

_____ Signs of drooling

_____ Tongue protrusion

_____ Sense of taste and smell

_____ Range of jaw motion during mouth opening

_____ Gag response

_____ Eye movements and pupil function

_____ Sensitivity of the face to touch

12. Select all of the following observations that are completed during examination of cranial nerves VIII–XII.

_____ Tongue symmetry and tone

_____ Sensitivity of the tongue to touch

_____ Elevation of the soft palate during phonation

_____ Tongue protrusion and other movements

_____ Sense of taste

_____ Voice quality during phonation

_____ Range of jaw motion during mouth opening phonation

_____ Hyolaryngeal elevation during a swallow

_____ Gag response

_____ Eye movements and pupil function

13. <u>TRUE</u> or <u>FALSE</u> (circle one): During the head and neck examination, the physician palpates the structures of the head and neck to check for masses as well as to determine increased size and reduced mobility of lymph nodes and the thyroid gland.

14. The two methods used by physicians to observe the hypopharyngeal and laryngeal structures during their examination include

    a. _____

    b. _____

15. Identify all of the following activities observed using flexible endoscopic examination.

    _____ Examination of the nasal passageways

    _____ Examination of the maxillary sinus

    _____ Velopharyngeal integrity and function during speech and swallowing

    _____ Base of tongue integrity and behavior during breathing, swallowing, and speech

    _____ Examination of taste and smell

    _____ Masses or tumors within the naso-, oro-, and laryngopharyngeal regions

    _____ Sensation of the oro- and hypopharyngeal structures

    _____ Oropharyngeal and hypopharyngeal clearance of boluses after a swallow

    _____ Tongue tip elevation during the oral phase

    _____ Vocal fold approximation during the swallow

    _____ Oropharyngeal and hypopharyngeal bolus residue after a swallow

3

Clinical Swallow Evaluation Questions

1. Describe the difference between a swallow screening versus a clinical swallow evaluation.

_____

_____

_____

2. Define the following swallow screening tests.

Water swallow tests:

_____

_____

_____

Toronto Bedside Swallowing Test (TOR-BSST):

_____

_____

_____

Cervical auscultation:

_____

_____

_____

Pulse oximetry:

_____

_____

_____

3. Select all of the correct indications for conducting a clinical swallow evaluation.

   _____ Pulmonary history suggestive of aspiration

   _____ The patient passed the swallow screening without swallowing complaints

   _____ Unexplained weight loss

   _____ Uneventful completion of an instrumental swallow imaging examination

   _____ Malnutrition or dehydration

   _____ Caregiver or patient concerns are expressed regarding swallowing problems

   _____ Dysarthria and a gurgly voice quality

   _____ The patient is unresponsive and on a ventilator

4. TRUE or FALSE (circle one): A clinical evaluation of swallowing should be bypassed when a patient is already scheduled to complete a videofluoroscopic evaluation of swallowing (i.e., dynamic swallow study [DSS]) or a flexible endoscopic evaluation of swallowing (FEES).

5. Identify five important features of normal deglutition.

   a. _____

   b. _____

   c. _____

   d _____

   e. _____

6. TRUE or FALSE (circle one): A clinical evaluation of swallowing can visualize the entire aerodigestive tract involved in deglutition.

7. TRUE or FALSE (circle one): A clinical evaluation of swallowing permits the clinician to determine the nature, severity, and likely contributions of the oral, pharyngeal, or esophageal components of deglutition to an individual's dysphagia.

8. Rate each of the following medical history and swallowing complaint items that may place an adult at risk for dysphagia versus not a risk factor for dysphagia.

A. At risk for dysphagia   **B. Not a risk factor for dysphagia**

_____ Weight gain

_____ Chronic obstructive pulmonary disorder

_____ Carotid artery surgery

_____ Non-English speaker

_____ Base-of-tongue cancer

_____ Developmental speech abnormality

_____ Tube feedings

_____ Normal oral diet

_____ Complete a meal within 30 min

_____ Choking on liquids

_____ Regurgitation of food 1 hr after eating

_____ Likes to talk during meals

_____ Sensation of a lump in the throat

_____ Appropriately responds to questions and follows instructions

_____ Food sticks in the throat at the level of the larynx

_____ Radiating pain down the left arm during running

_____ Gradual increase in sticking of food in the throat after 65 years of age

_____ Drooling

_____ Head tilting to assist in getting food to the throat to swallow

_____ Dysarthria

_____ Uncuffed trach tube in place

_____ Hearing loss

_____ Fed by caregiver

_____ Cerebral palsy

_____ Stroke

_____ Hiatal hernia

_____ Food residue in the oral sulci

_____ Poor dentition and oral hygiene

_____ Excessively dry mouth

_____ Prefers to eat meat and potatoes

_____ Has a twin

_____ Completed radiation therapy to the head or neck

_____ Poor vision

_____ Difficulty swallowing pills

9. List the supplies and equipment necessary for completing a clinical evaluation of swallowing.

_____

_____

_____

_____

10. Select all of the following that are included as components of a clinical evaluation of swallowing.

_____ Videofluoroscopic evaluation

_____ Medical and surgical history

_____ Past and current medications

_____ Swallowing history

_____ Penmanship during writing task

_____ Respiratory status assessment

_____ Physical examination of the oral mechanism

_____ Vision testing

_____ Evaluate articulatory precision and rate

_____ Sensation to pinprick on the arms

_____ Sensation to taste of sugar, salt, or lemon

_____ Assessment of patient cognitive status and alertness

_____ Hearing thresholds to pure tones

_____ Assess signs of aspiration during swallowing of food and liquid

_____ Oropharyngeal reflex testing

11. CLINICAL CASE CHALLENGE: Mr. Jones is 1 week poststroke affecting the left cortex and is in an acute care hospital. You have received a request to complete a clinical evaluation of swallowing to determine whether Mr. Jones should remain NPO (no food by mouth) or whether he can resume oral eating (PO). Upon entering the room, Mr. Jones is sitting upright in his bed and greets you, responding appropriately to your questions throughout your conversation. Mr. Jones tells you that he currently chokes on water when he drinks from a cup, but not when he drinks using a straw. As he talks, you note that he exhibits slight imprecise articulation of anterior lingual speech sounds (e.g., /t/, /d/, /n/, etc.). During tongue protrusion, you note that Mr. Jones's tongue deviates toward his right; however, his tongue appears symmetric and tone at rest during examination of the oral structures. The soft palate also appears symmetric and elevates bilaterally upon phonation of "ah." The symmetry of Mr. Jones's face appears to droop on the lower right side with the remainder of his face within normal limits for tone and symmetry. He exhibits the ability to wrinkle his forehead bilaterally; however, you observe that Mr. Jones is drooling from the right side of his mouth. You administer an ice chip and observe the Mr. Jones exhibits mild difficulty manipulating the ice chip and it falls into the pharynx triggering a choking episode.

a. Based on the observations described previously, identify at least two hypotheses you have at this point in the clinical evaluation.

_____

_____

_____

_____

_____

_____

b. Given the previously described findings, what additional clinical evaluation components would you administer? Provide a rationale for your response.

_____

_____

_____

_____

_____

_____

c. Given your charge to determine whether Mr. Jones can begin oral eating, consider whether the clinical evaluation of swallowing will suffice or whether you already have enough information to warrant additional testing. Provide a recommendation for whether additional testing is needed, including your rationale.

_____

_____

_____

_____

_____

_____

12. Practice completing a clinical evaluation of swallowing on a friend, family member, or fellow student. An extensive teaching-based form is included in this workbook to help you organize the sequence of information that needs to be gathered during this type of evaluation. Once you feel comfortable with the protocol, you will be ready to work with a patient under supervision by an expert in the area of adult-based dysphagia. Several of the components of this particular protocol overlap with clinical evaluation with pediatric populations; however, there are also significant differences.

Materials and Supplies Typically Needed:

Sugar packets, or sugar solution (10%)

Salt packets, or NaCl solution (10%)

Coffee, orange or lemon rind, chocolate, peppermint oil, or gum

Flashlight

Tongue depressor

Cotton swab

Timer or stopwatch

Gloves

Eyewear

Gauze pads

Paper cups

Straws

Spoons

Nasal mirror

Ice chips

Water

Applesauce

Saltine crackers or shortbread cookie

Stethoscope (for auscultation)

Patient Name: _____ Date: _____

Patient DOB: _____   Clinician: _____

Patient Weight: _____   Height: _____   Gender: Male   Female

A. Medical History	
Referral Source:	
Concern on Referral:	
Primary Patient Complaint:	
Date of Onset:	
Medications:	____ Antidepressant; ____ Antipsychotic; ____ Sedative; ____ Antihistamine; ____ Diuretic; ____ Mucosal anesthetic; ____ Anticholinergic (please list medications below):
Medical Diagnosis(es):	
Surgical History (include approximate dates):	
Related Medical History:	
Cardiac:	
Gastroenterology (GI):	
Pulmonary:	

Neurological:	
Otolaryngology (ENT):	
Dental:	
Speech-Language Pathology:	
Social/Family:	
Primary Language(s):	
Occupation:	
Hearing Status:	
Respiratory Status:	YES NO Ventilator dependent? YES NO Tracheostoma without tube? YES NO Tracheostomy tube (if yes, identify type: _____) ___ Cuffed ___ Uncuffed ___ Fenestrated ___ Passy Muir valve ___ Finger occluded Other pertinent information (e.g., duration of placement, progression in transitioning to independent breathing, hygiene status, etc.):

B. Patient Status and Observations	YES	NO
The patient is alert and oriented to time and place		
The patient is attentive and responds appropriately to questions		
The patient appears confused, disoriented, or unable to respond appropriately to questions		
The patient appears ___ lethargic ___ sedated ___ unresponsive		
The patient is cooperative		
The patient is uncooperative		
The patient is able to sit upright ___ independently ___ with assistance		

	YES	NO
The patient is unable to sit upright without assistance		
The patient is able to ambulate ___ independently ___ with assistance		
The patient is immobile ___ requires a wheelchair ___ is bedridden		
The patient is able to feed him/herself independently		
The patient requires adapted eating utensils or products to feed independently		
The patient is eating an oral diet ___ without modification ___ with modification or restriction		
The patient is not eating an oral diet ___ NG ___ NJ ___ PEG ___ TPN		
The patient is able to maintain oral hygiene ___ independently ___ with assistance		
The patient exhibits poor oral hygiene		
OTHER OBSERVATIONS:		

C. SIGNS AND SYMPTOMS:	YES	NO
Increased duration of meals		
Frequent or excessively dry mouth		
Coughing/choking associated with eating		
Food or pills get stuck (ask them to point to location):		
Food remains in the oral cavity or in pockets between the teeth and inside of the cheek(s) when eating		
Sensation of a lump in the throat		
Food or liquid come out of the nose		

	YES	NO
Food or liquid spill from the mouth while eating		
Feel a burning sensation		
Experiences heartburn, indigestion, or burning in the chest associated with eating		
Experiences a wet or gurgly voice quality associated with eating		
Experiences an increased body temperature or spikes a fever within an hour of eating a meal		
Difficulty swallowing liquids		
Difficulty swallowing thicker foods that are not solid, such as applesauce, mashed potatoes, or cooked vegetables		
Difficulty swallowing solid foods such as meat or raw vegetables		
Frequent throat clearing associated with eating		
Changes in sense of smell (describe):		
Changes in taste sensation (describe):		
Onset of eating and swallowing problems was ___ Sudden ___ Gradual (describe duration of onset):		
Swallowing problems occur during specific meals: ___ Breakfast ___ Lunch ___ Dinner ___ Snacks		
Swallowing problems occur during specific times of day: ___ Morning ___ Afternoon ___ Evening ___ Waken during the night		
OTHER SIGNS AND SYMPTOMS:		

Oropharyngeal Sensory Motor Examination Sense of Smell (CN I)

Ask the patient to close their eyes and tell you if and when they smell each of the following items (do not tell them what you are offering), and indicate those they correctly identified.

_____ Orange or lemon rind

_____ Coffee

_____ Chocolate

_____ Peppermint

Face and Lips (CN VII)

If asymmetric at rest, identify the abnormal facial quadrant using the diagram to the right:

<u>QUADRANT</u> **I   II   III   IV**

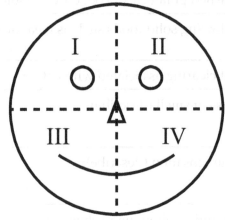

Describe abnormal appearance:

Sensory Motor Examination of the Oropharyngeal Mechanism for Eating						
FACE & LIPS (CN V & CN VII)	**YES**	**NO**	**L/R**	**ROM Impaired** (1 = mild, 2 = mod, 3 = severe)	**Strength Impaired** (1 = mild, 2 = mod, 3 = severe)	**Sensation Impaired** (1 = mild, 2 = mod, 3 = severe)
RESTING OBSERVATION						
The face is symmetric at rest:						
Lip tremor observed:						
Adequate lip closure at rest:						
MOVEMENT ASSESSMENT						
Lift the eyebrows, or try to look at the ceiling to wrinkle the forehead:						
Close eyelids tightly against resistance:						
Smile widely so that the teeth show:						
Pucker the lips as though kissing:						
Alternate smiling and puckering the lips as fast as possible for 7 s:						
Smack the lips:						
Frown while showing teeth (grimace):						
Puff out the cheeks and hold air in the mouth:						
Puff out the cheeks and hold air in the mouth against pressure applied to each cheek and then both cheeks:						
Move mouth from side to side:						
Say the sound "ooh" (lip rounding during speech):						
Say the sound "ee" (lip spreading during speech):						
Alternate saying "ooh ee ooh ee . . . " as quickly as possible for 7 s:						

FACE & LIPS (CN V & CN VII)	YES	NO	L/R	ROM Impaired (1 = mild, 2 = mod, 3 = severe)	Strength Impaired (1 = mild, 2 = mod, 3 = severe)	Sensation Impaired (1 = mild, 2 = mod, 3 = severe)
MOVEMENT ASSESSMENT						
Repeat the sound "puh" as quickly as possible for 5 s (5 to 7 syllables/s = norm for adults):						
Does the patient exhibit imprecise articulation of /p/?						
SENSORY ASSESSMENT						
Using a cotton ball or Q-tip, gently touch the 3 regions of the face supplied by CN V as well as the upper and lower lips and note any areas of reduced sensation:						
JAW & TONGUE (CN V, XII, VII, IX)	YES	NO	L/R	ROM Impaired (1 = mild, 2 = mod, 3 = severe)	Strength Impaired (1 = mild, 2 = mod, 3 = severe)	Sensation Impaired (1 = mild, 2 = mod, 3 = severe)
RESTING OBSERVATION						
Does the jaw appear symmetric at rest?						
Does the jaw exhibit a tremor?						
Does the jaw hang lower than normal?						
Is the patient edentulous?						
Does the patient have adequate and healthy dentition and oral hygiene?						
Does the patient exhibit poor oral hygiene and dentition status?						
Open the mouth widely—does the tongue appear symmetrical?						
Does the tongue exhibit fasciculations? (The tongue must be positioned at rest in the mouth for this observation.)						

JAW & TONGUE (CN V, XII, VII, IX)	YES	NO	L/R	ROM Impaired (1 = mild, 2 = mod, 3 = severe)	Strength Impaired (1 = mild, 2 = mod, 3 = severe)	Sensation Impaired (1 = mild, 2 = mod, 3 = severe)
RESTING OBSERVATION						
Does the tongue exhibit unilateral grooves, symmetric grooves, or furrows on the surface of the tongue evidencing atrophy?						
Does the tongue exhibit a scalloped appearance around the edges (impressions from teeth)?						
Does the tongue or other oral mucosa appear dry or exhibit signs of xerostomia?						
Does the tongue exhibit tremor in its rest position?						
Are there secretions or signs of pocketed food within the oral cavity or under the tongue?						
MOVEMENT ASSESSMENT						
Open mouth as wide as possible:						
Try to close your mouth against resistance:						
Try to open your mouth against resistance:						
Now move the jaw to each side (left and right):						
Open and close your mouth as quickly as possible for 7 s:						
Clench the jaw together (i.e., bite):						
Does the patient exhibit a normal occlusion during the bite? Or malocclusion (describe):						
Ask the patient to stick out their tongue and hold it for 2 s or more:						
Rapid repetitive lateral motion of the tongue between the left and right angles for 7 s (with mouth held open):						

JAW & TONGUE (CN V, XII, VII, IX)	YES	NO	L/R	ROM Impaired (1 = mild, 2 = mod, 3 = severe)	Strength Impaired (1 = mild, 2 = mod, 3 = severe)	Sensation Impaired (1 = mild, 2 = mod, 3 = severe)
MOVEMENT ASSESSMENT						
Rapid repetitive lateral motion of the tongue between the left and right cheeks for 7 s (with the mouth held open):						
Lick the periphery of the lips (along the vermilion border):						
With the mouth open, place the tongue tip behind the upper front teeth:						
With the mouth open, reach the tongue tip toward the nose:						
With the mouth open, place the tongue tip behind the lower front teeth:						
With the mouth open, reach the tongue tip toward the chin:						
Retract the tongue as far into the mouth as possible:						
Trace the tongue along the hard palate from behind the teeth to as far back as possible (with the mouth held open):						
Does the patient move the tongue without needing to move the jaw?						
Using a tongue blade, ask the patient to push the tongue tip against the tongue blade during tongue protrusion (i.e., against resistance):						
Ask the patient to push their tongue against the inside of their left cheek against the resistance of your finger. Repeat tongue lateral strength testing with the right cheek:						

JAW & TONGUE (CN V, XII, VII, IX)	YES	NO	L/R	ROM Impaired (1 = mild, 2 = mod, 3 = severe)	Strength Impaired (1 = mild, 2 = mod, 3 = severe)	Sensation Impaired (1 = mild, 2 = mod, 3 = severe)
MOVEMENT ASSESSMENT						
Using a tongue blade, apply pressure to the tongue dorsum and ask the patient to try to elevate his tongue tip against it:						
Using a tongue blade, apply pressure to the left and then right sides of the tongue and ask the patient to try to resist their tongue being moved:						
Repeat the sound "tuh" as rapidly as possible for 5 s (5–7 syllables/s = norm for adults):						
Repeat the sound "kuh" as rapidly as possible for 5 s (5–7 syllables/s = norm for adults):						
Repeat combinations of "puh tuh," "tuh kuh," and "puh tuh kuh" as rapidly as possible for 5 s (5–7 syllables/s = norm for adults):						
Does the patient exhibit imprecise articulation of /t/?						
Does the patient exhibit imprecise articulation of /k/?						
SENSORY ASSESSMENT						
Using a Q-tip, apply light touch to the posterior left and right sides of the tongue while the patient closes their eyes and raises their hand when they sense touch:						
Using a Q-tip, apply light touch to the anterior left and right sides of the tongue while the patient keeps their eyes closed and raises their hand when they sense touch:						

JAW & TONGUE (CN, V, XII, VII, IX)	YES	NO	L/R	ROM Impaired (1 = mild, 2 = mod, 3 = severe)	Strength Impaired (1 = mild, 2 = mod, 3 = severe)	Sensation Impaired (1 = mild, 2 = mod, 3 = severe)
SENSORY ASSESSMENT						
Apply the Q-tip to the hard palate and soft palate regions along the midline while the patient keeps their eyes closed and raises their hand when they sense touch:						
Using a Q-tip and while the patient keeps their eyes closed, place it in a solution of 10% NaCl (salt) and touch it to the left side of the patient's protruded tongue and wait to see if they signal tasting it, then test the right side of the tongue in the same way:						
Using a Q-tip and while the patient keeps their eyes closed, place it in a solution of 10% glucose (sugar) and touch it to the left side of the patient's protruded tongue and wait to see if they signal tasting it, then test the right side of the tongue in the same way:						
HARD/SOFT PALATE, PHARYNX, LARYNX (CN, IX, X, XI)	YES	NO	L/R	ROM Impaired (1 = mild, 2 = mod, 3 = severe)	Strength Impaired (1 = mild, 2 = mod, 3 = severe)	Sensation Impaired (1 = mild, 2 = mod, 3 = severe)
RESTING OBSERVATION						
Do the palatal arches appear symmetrical?						
Does the hard palate appear intact (if no, note cleft side, etc.)?						
Does the vault of the hard palate appear normal (if no, note abnormality)?						
Does the soft palate appear symmetric?						

HARD/SOFT PALATE, PHARYNX, LARYNX (CN, IX, X, XI)	YES	NO	L/R	ROM Impaired (1 = mild, 2 = mod, 3 = severe)	Strength Impaired (1 = mild, 2 = mod, 3 = severe)	Sensation Impaired (1 = mild, 2 = mod, 3 = severe)
RESTING OBSERVATION						
Does the soft palate exhibit rhythmic or arrhythmic movements characteristic of a myoclonus?						
Do you hear audible inhalation (i.e., stridor) or wheezing?						
MOVEMENT ASSESSMENT						
Does the palate elevate symmetrically during sustained phonation of "ah" (ask the patient to open their mouth wide—you may need to use a tongue blade to hold the tongue down to get a good look at the soft palate)?						
Say the sound "ah" loudly (not yelling, however) 5 times and note soft palate elevation consistency and symmetry:						
Do you observe lateral or posterior pharyngeal wall constriction during sustained or repeated production of "ah"?						
Is the patient's resonance normal? Or do you hear hypernasality or hyponasality?						
Does the voice sound hoarse?						
Does the voice sound excessively breathy?						
Does the voice sound wet and gurgly?						
If the voice sounds wet and gurgly, ask the patient to clear their throat and sustain the sound "ah" again. Does it still sound wet and gurgly?						

HARD/SOFT PALATE, PHARYNX, LARYNX (CN, IX, X, XI)	YES	NO	L/R	ROM Impaired (1 = mild, 2 = mod, 3 = severe)	Strength Impaired (1 = mild, 2 = mod, 3 = severe)	Sensation Impaired (1 = mild, 2 = mod, 3 = severe)
MOVEMENT ASSESSMENT						
Ask the patient to take a deep breath and then bear down while holding their breath—can they hold their breath? Or do they exhibit air leakage during this task?						
Ask the patient to hold their breath for as long as possible and time how long they can do this (30–60 s is average):						
Ask the patient to perform a sharp cough—rate the cough using the following descriptors:						
a. The cough was brisk with sharp, hard onset of voicing followed by a strong audible exhalation.						
b. Mildly weak cough						
c. Moderately weak cough						
d. Severely weak cough						
e. Unable to produce a voluntary cough						
Do you feel elevation of the larynx during a dry swallow?						
SENSORY ASSESSMENT						
Does the patient gag or show sensitivity to the touch of a tongue blade or Q-tip to the posterior 1/3 of the tongue?						
Does the patient gag or show sensitivity to the touch of a tongue blade to the posterior oropharynx?						

Respiratory Assessment

i) Record the number of breaths taken per second: _____ (norm = 12–16)

ii) Ability to complete a dry swallow during quiet breathing without discomfort:

____ YES ____ NO   (if no, describe the breathing pattern relative to swallowing)

iii) Duration of breath holding (instructed previously): _____

Food Assessment

If the patient has been NPO before now, make sure they have completed oral hygiene cleaning before administering anything orally. If the patient has been eating orally, ask them to bring food they are currently eating or observe them during their mealtime.

FOOD OR LIQUID ADMINISTERED	Voice quality remains clear? (Y/N)	Timely onset of swallow? (Y/N)	Cough response observed? (Y/N)	If cough observed, was it effective in clearing the bolus? (Y/N)	Evidence of nasal regurgitation? (Y/N)	Was the bolus adequately controlled during the trial? (Y/N)	Compensatory behaviors observed due to eating difficulties? (Y/N)	OTHER OBSERVATIONS:
Ice chips								
1 tsp of water								
3 oz of water								
Typical large sip of water from a cup (~10–20 mL)								
Sequential swallows using a straw								
1 tsp of applesauce								
1 tsp of pudding (e.g., Jell-O pudding cups)								
A bit of saline cracker or cookie								
FILL IN OBSERVATION OF TYPICAL FOODS EATEN:								

Recommendations:

_____   Regular PO diet (unrestricted diet)

Diet Modification

Oral versus nonoral nutrition and hydration:

_____   PO with modification or dietary restrictions (specify):

_____   Free water protocol between meals only (requires oral hygiene)

_____   Ice chips

_____   Medication form may require modification (e.g., pill, liquid)

_____   **IDDSI 0 (THIN)** = Can drink through any type of teat/nipple, cup, or straw as appropriate for age and skills. Liquids flow like water (i.e., fast flow).

_____   **IDDSI 1 (SLIGHTLY THICK)** = Predominantly used in the pediatric population as a thickened drink that reduces the speed of flow but is still able to flow through an infant teat/nipple. Thicker than water, but flows through a straw, syringe, or teat/nipple with similar thickness to commercially available "antiregurgitation" (AR) infant formula.

_____   **IDDSI 2 (MILDLY THICK)** = Flows or pours quickly from a spoon but can be sipped. Effort is required to drink this thickness through a standard bore straw (i.e., .209 in. or 5.3 mm diameter). Suitable if tongue control is slightly reduced.

_____   **IDDSI 3 (MODERATELY THICK/LIQUIDIZED)** = Can be drunk from a cup but requires some effort to suck through a standard bore straw (i.e., .209 in. or 5.3 mm diameter). Cannot be piped, layered, or moulded on a plate and cannot be eaten on a fork because it drips slowly in dollops through the prongs. Can be eaten with a spoon. No oral processing or chewing required and is a smooth texture without "bits." Allows more time for oral control and can be used when there is pain on swallowing.

_____   **IDDSI 4 (PUREED/EXTREMELY THICK)** = Usually eaten with a spoon, but can also be eaten with a fork. Cannot be drunk from a cup or sucked through a straw. Does not require chewing and can be piped, layered, or molded. Shows slow movement under gravity, but cannot be poured. Falls off a spoon in a single spoonful when tilted and continues to hold shape on a plate. No lumps and is not sticky. No biting or chewing is required making this a good level for those with missing teeth, poorly fitting dentures, or pain on chewing or swallowing.

_____   **IDDSI 5 (MINCED & MOIST)** = Can be eaten with a fork, spoon, or chopsticks (with good hand control). Can be scooped or shaped on a plate with small lumps visible within the food (pediatric = 2-mm lump size; adult = 4-mm lump size). Lumps are easy to squash with the tongue. Biting is not required and chewing is minimal. Tongue force is required to move the bolus and works with individuals identified with missing teeth, poorly fitting dentures, or pain or fatigue on chewing.

_____ **IDDSI 6 (SOFT & BITE-SIZED)** = Can be eaten with a fork, spoon, or chopsticks. Food can be mashed/broken down and does not require a knife to cut. Biting is not required, but chewing is required before swallowing. Bite-sized pieces should be as appropriate for size and oral processing skills (pediatric = 8-mm pieces; adult = 15-mm or 1.5-cm size pieces). Tongue force and control of the bolus is required to move the bolus for swallowing and can be used with those with missing teeth, poorly fitting dentures, or pain or fatigue on chewing.

_____ **IDDSI 7 (REGULAR)** = Normal, everyday foods of various textures that are developmentally and age appropriate. NO TEXTURE RESTRICTIONS. Any method may be used to eat these foods and a range of sizes can be eaten (pediatric = < or > 8-mm pieces; adult = < or > 15 mm or 1.5 cm). Includes hard, tough, chewy, fibrous, stringy, dry, crispy, crunchy, or crumbly bits and foods that contain pips, seeds, pith inside skin, husks, or bones. Also includes dual and mixed consistency foods and liquids.

_____ NPO (Nil per os = nothing per mouth)

  _____ With supplemental oral intake (specify):

  _____ Without supplemental oral intake

Compensatory Strategies

Positional Strategies:

☐ Chin tuck (i.e., neck flexion)

☐ Head turn right versus left (select one)

☐ Lean or tilt to the right versus left (select one)

☐ OTHER:

Swallowing Maneuvers:

☐ Multiple swallows per bolus

☐ Breath hold prior to swallow

☐ Mendelsohn maneuver

☐ Effortful swallow

☐ Audible exhalation after the swallow

☐ Supraglottic Swallow

☐ Super Supraglottic Swallow

☐ OTHER:

Adaptations or Compensations:

☐ Assistance with feeding

☐ Verbal cues

☐ Food placement on plate

☐ Complete feeding assistance by other person

☐ Adaptive feeding device or method (refer to occupational therapy)

☐ Alternate liquids with food

☐ Reduce rate of eating

☐ Add moisture to dry foods (e.g., gravy, condiments, etc.)

☐ Temperature of food (select specifications of temperature):

    ☐ Ice chips

    ☐ Cold foods

    ☐ Warm foods

    ☐ Hot foods

☐ Small and more frequent meals

☐ Oral tongue/finger sweep

☐ OTHER:

INDIRECT TREATMENT:

Progressive resistive tongue exercises

☐ Shaker exercises

☐ Masako method

☐ Lee Silverman Voice Treatment

☐ Expiratory muscle strengthening exercises

☐ Neuromuscular electrical stimulation

☐ Tongue strengthening and ROM exercises

☐ Lip strengthening exercises

☐ Jaw strengthening and ROM exercises

☐ Hawk exercise

☐ Neck flexion against resistance in upright position

☐ Jaw depression against resistance in upright position

☐ Biofeedback approaches (e.g., surface EMG, FEES, etc.)

☐ OTHER:

ADDITIONAL TESTING NEEDED:

☐ Gastroenterology consultation

☐ Neurology consultation

☐ Otolaryngology consultation

☐ Occupational therapy consultation

☐ Physical therapy consultation

☐ Dietitian consultation

☐ Home health referral

☐ Social work assistance

☐ Flexible endoscopic evaluation of swallowing and sensory testing

☐ Pharyngeal manometry

☐ Radiology referral:

    ☐ Chest X-ray (with physician input)

    ☐ MRI (with physician input)

    ☐ CT (with physician input)

    ☐ Scintigraphy (with physician input)

    ☐ OTHER:

4

Endoscopy in Assessing and Treating Dysphagia Questions

1. Select all of the following that identify an advantage of using endoscopy for evaluation of dysphagia.

    _____ The patient needs a same-day bedside evaluation.

    _____ The patient aspirates during the swallow.

    _____ A swallowing evaluation in the clinic is needed.

    _____ Need to rule out impaired mobility and range of motion of pharyngeal anatomy.

    _____ The patient's cricopharyngeus does not relax during the swallow.

    _____ There are concerns regarding radiation exposure for the patient.

    _____ The patient has reduced hyolaryngeal excursion during the swallow.

    _____ Need to test the foods typically eaten by the patient.

    _____ Need to observe secretions within the pharynx and their buildup over several swallows.

    _____ Need to evaluate problems experienced during the swallow to determine the cause.

    _____ Laryngeal and pharyngeal sensitivity are questioned and need evaluation.

    _____ Need to observe the coordination of bolus flow and airway protection.

    _____ The patient has a bleeding disorder.

    _____ Would like to use biofeedback during swallowing maneuvers.

    _____ Need to directly evaluate the impact of swallowing maneuvers and positions.

    _____ The patient predominantly has an oral-stage dysphagia.

2. Using endoscopy to evaluate the swallow will allow direct observation of aspiration when it occurs under these conditions.
    a. Aspiration prior to the swallow
    b. Aspiration during the swallow
    c. Aspiration after the swallow
    d. All of the above are correct.
    e. Only (a) and (c) are possible.

3. The definition of laryngeal penetration is that the bolus

   a. is observed on the laryngeal surface of the epiglottis but does not enter the laryngeal vestibule.

   b. is observed to penetrate the laryngeal aditus into the laryngeal vestibule and below the vocal folds.

   c. is observed to penetrate the laryngeal aditus into the laryngeal vestibule but does not penetrate below the vocal folds.

   d. All of the above.

4. The flexible endoscopic evaluation of swallowing (FEES) test evaluates the function of all of these valves EXCEPT the

   a. velopharynx.

   b. larynx.

   c. pharyngoesophageal segment.

   d. lips.

5. The following is an example of a task that tests the function of the velopharyngeal port during closure.

   a. Sniffing

   b. Sustained phonation of /s/

   c. Sustaining the sound /m/

   d. Production of a slow nasal inhalation and a slow nasal exhalation

6. TRUE or FALSE (circle one): During evaluation of the velopharynx, attention should only be directed at soft palate movement, which should elevate during production of speech sounds.

7. All of the following can be done to assess pharyngeal musculature EXCEPT

   a. sustain phonation of /a/ (pronounced "ah").

   b. sustain phonation of /i/ (pronounced "ee") while performing an upward pitch glide.

   c. touch the epiglottis or arytenoid mucosa with the scope tip.

   d. retract and protrude the tongue and observe base of tongue and posterior pharyngeal wall movements.

8. Which of the following can be done to assess laryngeal function and airway protection?

   a. Sustain phonation of /i/ (pronounced "ee") for several seconds

   b. Perform a sniff and then say /i/ to observe the range of vocal fold mobility

   c. Sustain phonation of /i/ while producing upward and downward pitch glides

   d. Observe vocal fold and laryngeal closure during breath holding

   e. Touch the tip of the scope to the arytenoid or vocal fold mucosa to test laryngeal sensitivity to touch

   f. All of the above.

9. In an individual who has not been eating food by mouth and is observed to have buildup of secretions upon imaging of the pharynx, the first swallowing task recommended is

   a. the ice chip protocol.

   b. swallowing of applesauce.

   c. swallowing of a 20-cc bolus of water with green food coloring.

   d. swallowing of orange juice.

10. One method that can be used during FEES to test the oral stage of deglutition is to

    a. have the patient complete sequential swallows.

    b. ask the patient to hold a liquid bolus in the oral cavity to the count of three before initiating the swallow.

    c. complete three sniffs.

    d. None of the above.

11. An important observation when residue is seen on the surface of the vocal folds or food spills into the larynx is whether

    a. the patient spontaneously coughs or throat clears.

    b. the patient can clear the material from the larynx on command.

    c. the bolus passes below the vocal folds without a reflexive cough.

    d. All of the above.

12. Number the following FEES tasks in the recommended sequence (from 1 to 6) in which they should be performed during an evaluation.

_____ Test positional, compensational, and swallowing maneuver techniques and observation of impact

_____ Administration of mechanically soft boluses

_____ Administration of a small liquid bolus

_____ Examination of the pharyngeal anatomy and movements

_____ Administration of solid foods, including mixed consistencies

_____ Administration of increasingly larger liquid boluses

13. TRUE or FALSE (circle one): It is important to use a generous amount of topical anesthesia to ensure the comfort of the patient during completion of the FEES evaluation.

14. TRUE or FALSE (circle one): The American Speech-Language-Hearing Association (ASHA) deems completion of FEES to be within the scope of practice for speech-language pathologists (SLPs). ASHA is the final authority on whether SLPs can or cannot complete a FEES in their work setting.

15. Flexible endoscopic evaluation of swallowing and sensory testing (FEESST) is different from FEES in that it

    a. entails the use of endoscopy to test deglutition.

    b. incorporates sensory testing of the pharynx and larynx.

    c. entails evaluation of the oral stage of deglutition.

    d. involves imaging of the esophagus.

16. Watch Video 4–1. FEESPT1 on the PluralPlus Companion Website. Select all of the following that are observed during this video.

_____ Secretions pooling on the vocal folds

_____ Buildup of secretions in the left piriform sinus

_____ Inadequate vocal fold approximation for phonation of /i/

_____ Immobility of the right vocal fold

_____ Absent movement or constriction of the pharyngeal walls

_____ Increased size of the left ventricular fold such that it obstructs most of the left vocal fold view

17. Which of the following occurred during breath holding during the FEES exam shown in Video 4–2. FEESPT2 on the Companion Website?

a. Exhalation during regurgitation evidenced by bubbling

b. Closure of the larynx during breath holding

c. Regurgitation of a green bolus into the hypopharynx

d. All of the above.

5

Barium Radiographic Evaluation of the Pharynx and Esophagus Questions

1. Define the following radiographic procedures.

   a. Cineradiography:

   _____

   _____

   b. Videofluoroscopy:

   _____

   _____

   c. Ultrasound:

   _____

   _____

   d. Computed tomography:

   _____

   _____

   e. Magnetic resonance imaging:

   _____

   _____

2. The oropharyngeal swallow is completed in _____ second(s) or less making six frames per second of rapid sequence filming <u>ADEQUATE</u> or <u>INADEQUATE</u> (circle one) for capturing adequate sampling for analysis.

3. Exposure to radiation is considered to be _____ throughout the lifetime. Thus, the National Council for Radiation Protection (NCRP) and the International Atomic Energy Association (IAEA) state that there <u>IS</u> or <u>IS NOT</u> (circle one) a safe dose of radiation.

4. All of the following are considered units of radiation EXCEPT

    a. sieverts.

    b. rads.

    c. hertz.

    d. gray.

5. Select all of the following factors that affect radiation dose exposure during a radiographic procedure.

    _____ Peak voltage across the X-ray tube (kVp)

    _____ Tube current × exposure time (milliampere seconds, mAs)

    _____ Wearing jewelry or glasses

    _____ Image field size

    _____ Source distance to the skin surface

    _____ Clothing material such as cotton versus leather

    _____ Source distance to the detector

    _____ Use of a grid

    _____ Metal fillings versus soft filling materials in the teeth

    _____ Screening time in advance of recording

6. All of the following statements regarding radiation exposure are true EXCEPT

    a. One chest X-ray = 0.01 mSv of radiation.

    b. A transatlantic flight from the United States = 0.04 mSV of radiation.

    c. A fluoroscopic swallowing study = 0.04 to 1 mSv of radiation.

    d. All of the above are true.

7. TRUE or FALSE (circle one): A videofluoroscopic evaluation of swallowing (i.e., dynamic swallow study) should be completed when information is needed to determine underlying problems with eating associated with the oral, pharyngeal, and/or esophageal stages.

8. All of the following statements regarding a videofluoroscopic evaluation of swallowing are true EXCEPT

   a. The patient can be examined in the lateral and the anterior–posterior planes.

   b. The lateral view is always completed first.

   c. It is the same as an esophagram.

   d. This method allows evaluation of aspiration occurring prior to, during, or after completion of the swallow.

9. Videofluoroscopic views are completed in the anterior–posterior plane of view to

   a. determine symmetries or asymmetries in bolus pathway and clearance.

   b. evaluate the function of the velopharynx.

   c. evaluate tongue movements associated with propulsion of the bolus into the pharynx from the oral cavity.

   d. None of the above; the anterior–posterior plane of view is rarely used or useful.

10. TRUE or FALSE (circle one): Silent aspiration is best evaluated during a clinical evaluation of swallowing rather than by using videofluoroscopy.

11. Videofluoroscopy allows quantification of the following measurements that cannot be made using flexible endoscopic evaluation of swallowing (FEES) EXCEPT

    a. hyolaryngeal displacement.

    b. pharyngoesophageal segment opening during the swallow.

    c. total pharyngeal transit time.

    d. degree of pharyngeal constriction during the swallow.

12. Upon completion of evaluation of the oropharyngeal portion of deglutition, a screening of the _____ can be completed. This is typically done during swallowing of a _____ cc bolus of liquid barium. This screen follows the bolus all the way to the _____. In addition to the liquid bolus, a 13-mm barium _____ is administered and followed from the oral cavity to the _____. This portion of the screening has a sensitivity and specificity of _____% for most esophageal problems.

13. The indentation observed on the left side of the radiograph shown in Figure 5–7 in the textbook is caused by the _____, and just below the same level, another indentation is observed and caused by the left _____.

14. Define these terms.

    a. Reflux:

    _____

    _____

    b. Trendelenburg position:

    _____

    _____

    c. Valsalva maneuver:

    _____

    _____

    d. Secondary peristalsis:

    _____

    _____

    e. Tertiary esophageal contractions:

    _____

    _____

6

Dynamic Fluoroscopic Swallow Study: Swallow Evaluation With Videofluoroscopy Questions

1. All of the following are possible reasons for completing a dynamic swallow study (DSS) EXCEPT to

   a. identify risks to respiratory/pulmonary health.

   b. identify risks to nutrition/hydration health.

   c. monitor an individual while he/she eats a meal.

   d. determine appropriate behavioral, surgical, or medical intervention.

   e. determine changes in disease or condition over time.

   f. determine changes in deglutition from pre- to posttreatment.

2. TRUE or FALSE (circle one): Dynamic swallow studies are often completed for the sole reason of observing whether there is a presence or absence of aspiration.

3. Select all of the following descriptions considered to be limitations of using videofluoroscopy (Dynamic Swallow Study [DSS]) to assess and manage dysphagia.

   _____ Radiation exposure limits testing duration to less than 5 min

   _____ Can observe the physiology underlying abnormal deglutition

   _____ Utilizes a standard protocol rather than observation of a typical meal

   _____ Images the oral, pharyngeal, and esophageal stages

   _____ Cannot test sensation of tissues

   _____ Can observe the timing of aspiration relative to the swallow

   _____ Can observe the location of residue after the swallow

   _____ Implementation of radiopaque contrast boluses

   _____ Individual must sit upright and be mobile

4. Identify information that is important to obtain prior to completing a DSS to determine the risk factors of the patient for aspiration and other forms of dysphagia.

   a. _____

   _____

   b. _____

   _____

c. _____

_____

d. _____

_____

5. All of the following are examples of the advantage of using a standard DSS protocol (select all that apply).

_____ So that each patient's performance on the DSS can be compared with those of others

_____ To reduce the need for the clinician to address problems that arise or to investigate effectiveness of interventional methods with the patient during the procedure

_____ To compare performance on the DSS over time or from pre- to posttreatment

_____ To ensure consistency in DSS performance across clinicians

_____ To enhance the opportunity for reimbursement for the DSS procedure

_____ To compare performance on different types of tests of deglutition (e.g., FEES, manometry)

6. DSS views in the lateral plane of view ideally should include views of these structures.

_____

_____

_____

7. DSS views in the anterior–posterior (A/P) plane of view allow all of the following EXCEPT

a. measurement of pharyngeal transit time.

b. assessment of symmetry of bolus movement.

c. vocal fold movement.

d. symmetry of hypopharyngeal residue.

e. screening of the esophageal stage of deglutition.

8. TRUE or FALSE (circle one): A DSS is ideally completed on an individual in the supine position to eliminate the assistance of gravity in helping the bolus move through the pharynx.

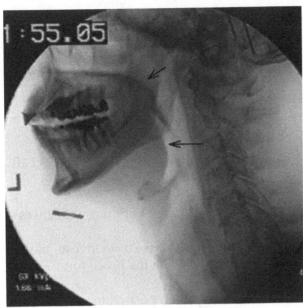

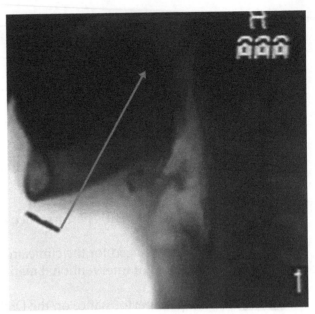

A   **B**

9. Figure A/B (circle one) is an ideal example of image acquisition during a dynamic swallow study with a fully visible oral cavity, pharynx, larynx, trachea, and pharyngoesophageal segment (PES). Figure A/B (circle one) is an example of poor visibility of the oral cavity, nasopharynx, and oropharynx. TRUE/FALSE (circle one): The image example of poor structural visibility is due to poor positioning of the patient.

10. Match the following variables with their correct description regarding their potential influence on patient performance or DSS success.

_____ Position of the patient/upper airway structures

_____ Postural stability/flexibility

_____ Respiratory sufficiency

_____ Stamina and endurance

_____ Lubrication

_____ Bolus characteristics

_____ Competing behaviors and states

_____ Environment

_____ Adaptability

_____ Imaging views

A. Mrs. Smith reported dryness as a side effect of her medications. During her DSS, difficulty clearing the cookie bolus from her oral cavity was demonstrated through multiple lingual initiations of bolus transit with bolus residue in the valleculae after completion of her swallow.

B. Mr. Jones is diagnosed with chronic obstructive pulmonary disease (COPD) and arrives using oxygen and with a rapid rate of respiration (i.e., 30 breaths per min). He is observed to initiate his swallow in a timely manner on thin liquids; however, his airway closure appears incomplete and opens as the bolus reaches the upper esophageal sphincter (UES), resulting in laryngeal penetration and aspiration of the liquid bolus.

C. Jimmy is a 7-year-old boy diagnosed with cerebral palsy and is in a wheelchair. His arms are spastically maintained in a flexed position and his torso and head position are maintained in an extended position with a head tilt laterally and toward the right. Due to Jimmy's positioning during swallowing, the right side of the pharynx appeared compressed and bolus clearance was predominantly through the left side of the pharynx. The head and neck structures were at an oblique angle during image acquisition.

D. Tammy demonstrated aspiration on thin liquid bolus trials, but no aspiration during swallows of nectar-thick liquids. Paste bolus trials appeared to clear well, but the cookie bolus was associated with residue in the vallecular and piriform sinuses.

E. Jon is a 3-year-old boy with a history of a posterior laryngeal cleft associated with aspiration during the swallow. His surgeon requested a swallow study to determine whether surgical correction was successful in closing the posterior larynx. Jon refused to drink or eat any of the testing materials for his DSS because he was more interested in the imaging equipment and radiology technician than eating.

F. Georgia was extremely fearful to swallow food since suffering an airway obstruction 1 month ago. She agreed to swallow liquid bolus trials during the DSS, but exhibited prolonged holding of paste and cookie bolus materials in her oral cavity and eventually spit them into a cup due to her fear of having another obstructive airway event.

G. Mr. Smith underwent a cervical neck fusion and reported onset of difficulty swallowing afterward. He was observed to exhibit laryngeal penetration with risk of aspiration during swallowing; however, implementation of neck flexion (i.e., chin tuck) was difficult due to his reduced neck flexibility.

H. Jack was post left glossectomy and demonstrated that he usually placed food on the right posterior tongue region and then tilted his head back to facilitate transit into the pharynx for swallowing.

I. Claire showed normal swallow function on her first two swallow trials, but gradually worsened as the DSS testing progressed. She reported that she often experiences this pattern during meals and needs to rest within a few minutes of initiating a meal, but can resume eating for short periods of time after resting.

J. Lou complained that solid foods would stick in his throat and this has worsened gradually over time. During lateral views of his DSS, bolus residue was observed at the level of the arytenoids in the pharynx. During A/P views, it was discovered that Lou had a left-sided diverticulum where residue collected, but would eventually empty after a second or third dry swallow.

11. Check all of the following items considered to be reasons for completing a standard protocol during DSS testing.

_____ Enables comparison of findings from pre- to posttreatment

_____ Enables comparison of findings to normative data

_____ Provides excessive radiation exposure to patients

_____ Improves testing consistency between and within clinicians and institutions

_____ Can be used to force patients to eat something they don't like

_____ Reduces radiation exposure due to the efficiency with which information is gathered

12. <u>TRUE</u> or <u>FALSE</u> (circle one): A metal ring or round object of a known diameter is secured on the midline under the chin of the individual undergoing a DSS so that completion of calibrated measures can be made of the DSS recordings.

13. Number the following items in their general recommended sequence during a DSS evaluation with an adult.

LATERAL VIEW:

_____ 20-cc bolus of liquid barium

_____ 1/4 of a shortbread cookie with paste barium

_____ 3-cc bolus of liquid barium

_____ 60-cc liquid barium via straw drinking

_____ 1-cc bolus of liquid barium

_____ 3-cc paste barium

A/P VIEW:

_____ 3-cc paste barium

_____ 13-mm barium capsule

_____ 20-cc liquid barium

14. All of the following are methods used to complete a DSS in the lateral view in infants EXCEPT

    a. sucking on a nipple or pacifier with a trace amount of barium contrast on it.

    b. drinking undiluted barium contrast liquid from a bottle during a suck-swallow sequence.

    c. drinking half sterilized water and half liquid barium during a suck-swallow sequence.

    d. chewing and swallowing a quarter of a shortbread cookie with paste barium.

15. TRUE or FALSE (circle one): The entire DSS protocol must be completed by every individual tested.

16. TRUE or FALSE (circle one): In the situation where continued administration of boluses appears too risky, modified speech tasks that target structural movements important to swallowing can be implemented to assess linguapalatal, velopharyngeal, and laryngeal valving and cough effectiveness.

17. Compensation and facilitation strategies include

    a. changing the effects of gravity on bolus flow.

    b. changing the size and relation between pharyngeal spaces and structures.

    c. increasing effort to modify swallowing gesture timing, range, and magnitude/force.

    d. All of the above.

18. Identify all of the following strategies that might be used to compensate for inadequate oral cavity function and safety.

    _____ Repeated swallows per bolus

    _____ Modified bolus consistency

    _____ Modified bolus volume

    _____ Prolonged maximum hyolaryngeal elevation

    _____ Modified bolus placement within the oral cavity

    _____ Bypassing the oral cavity with a syringe or catheter

    _____ Palatal lift prosthetic device

    _____ Preswallow breath holding

    _____ Head/neck flexion

    _____ Prolonged laryngeal closure after the swallow

19. Identify all of the following compensatory strategies that might be used with a 3-month-old infant exhibiting struggle and choking when drinking liquid from a standard nipple.

_____ Place the infant in neck flexion during swallowing

_____ Ask the infant to hold his/her breath before taking in a liquid bolus to swallow

_____ Use a nipple with a slower rate of release

_____ Limit the infant to consuming thicker bolus consistencies

_____ Position the infant in a less supine position during feeding

_____ Recommend tube feedings and place the infant on NPO (nil per oral) status

7

DSS: A Systematic Approach to Analysis and Interpretation Questions

1. Systematic analysis of deglutition using videofluoroscopy should cover all of the following EXCEPT

    a. evaluation of the timing and movement of oropharyngeal structures.

    b. evaluation of the competency of the oropharyngeal valves.

    c. evaluation of how well the patient progressed through her/his typical meal.

    d. variations in oropharyngeal swallow performance across consistency and volume contexts.

2. Effectiveness of deglutition can be affected by all of the following EXCEPT

    a. position of the torso, head, and neck.

    b. fluoroscopic frame size.

    c. flexibility of the upper body, head, and neck.

    d. respiratory insufficiency.

    e. impaired salivary production.

    f. bolus consistency and volume.

3. TRUE or FALSE (circle one): Measuring the timing of structural gestures and comparing them with the timing of bolus positions can reveal breakdowns in gesture sequences that contribute to the observed dysphagia.

4. TRUE or FALSE (circle one): Observation of the timing and range of movement of structures can elucidate between dysphagia associated with impaired movement, impaired coordination of movement, or the position of the bolus relative to structural movements during pharyngeal transit.

5. Impaired function of the linguapalatal valve may be reflected by

    a. oral transit time.

    b. oral preparation time.

    c. poor bolus containment in the oral cavity during oral preparation.

    d. nasal regurgitation.

6. Poor oral clearance of a bolus may be due to all of the following EXCEPT

 a. postradiation xerostomia.

 b. reduced hyolaryngeal excursion.

 c. reduced oral sensation.

 d. impaired tongue mobility and strength.

7. TRUE or FALSE (circle one): Displacement and duration of linguapalatal valving are the oral chamber events typically measured during a DSS evaluation.

8. Assessment of the competency of linguapalatal valving during deglutition is best conducted

 a. with the head and neck in a neutral position.

 b. with the head and neck in a flexed or extended position.

 c. in an upright position with the head rotated to the same side as hand dominance.

 d. with an open-jaw position.

9. Oropharyngeal transit time is defined to begin when the _____ valve begins to open (when the soft palate and tongue separate) and ends when the head of the bolus passes the _____.

10. Prolonged oropharyngeal transit time may be due to

 a. insufficient linguapalatal valving.

 b. mucosal dryness that slows bolus movement.

 c. oral or oropharyngeal structural abnormalities that impede bolus flow.

 d. altered gravitational effects due to head/neck and body position.

 e. All of the above.

 f. None of the above.

11. During deglutition, the structures of the upper airway must alternate between their involvement in _____ and _____ protection during the oropharyngeal swallow. The valves involved in directing the bolus to and through the oropharynx are the _____ and _____ valves. The valve involved in protecting the airway from bolus entry is the _____ valve.

12. The epiglottis

    a. is an important obstruction to divert bolus flow around the larynx through the lateral pharyngeal gutters.

    b. can serve as an obstruction to bolus clearance when it does not retrovert during the swallow.

    c. is vital to prevention of aspiration during the swallow.

    d. Both (a) and (b) are correct, but (c) is not.

    e. All of the above are correct.

13. TRUE or FALSE (circle one): Nasal regurgitation is primarily a sign that the soft palate did not elevate, as pharyngeal constriction is a minor contributor to velopharyngeal valving.

14. TRUE or FALSE (circle one): Velopharyngeal valving is controlled by the same neural pathways as speech, making it likely that nasal regurgitation is expected when individuals exhibit hypernasality during speech production.

15. TRUE or FALSE (circle one): The presence of the bolus in the hypopharynx (laryngopharynx) is associated with increased risk for aspiration.

16. Hypopharyngeal transit time

    a. begins when the bolus head passes the mandibular ramus.

    b. begins when the bolus head exits the valleculae.

    c. ends when the head of the bolus passes through the pharyngoesophageal segment (PES).

    d. ends when the tail of the bolus clears the PES.

    e. Both (b) and (d) are correct.

    f. Both (a) and (c) are correct.

    g. None of the above statements are correct.

17. Prolonged hypopharyngeal transit time can be explained by all of the following EXCEPT

    a. impaired coordination of bolus arrival in the hypopharynx with onset of hypopharyngeal structural movements/gestures associated with onset of the swallow.

    b. reduced or weak sequential constriction of the hypopharyngeal space resulting in poor bolus clearance.

    c. anatomic changes in the hypopharynx resulting in bolus obstruction.

    d. the presence of a Schatzki A-ring.

    e. All of the above.

18. The reason hypopharyngeal residue increases risk of aspiration is because

_____

_____

19. The presence of some residue after a swallow <u>IS</u> or <u>IS NOT</u> (circle one) normal, especially in elderly patients.

20. The best method for determination of the site associated with incomplete hypopharyngeal clearing is to identify the point of maximum _____ during the swallow. Symmetry of pharyngeal constriction is best evaluated in the _____ plane of view during videofluoroscopy.

21. Reduced or absent _____ excursion may be associated with hypopharyngeal residue related to incomplete opening of the _____.

22. Supraglottic penetration of bolus material
    a. is considered a risk for increased aspiration when it occurs frequently.
    b. is considered a risk for increased aspiration when the bolus is not extruded from the laryngeal vestibule during the swallow.
    c. is considered to be the same as aspiration when it is observed during the swallow.
    d. Only (a) and (c) are correct.
    e. All of the above are correct.

23. Select all of the following statements that are true regarding aspiration relative to laryngeal closure during deglutition.

_____ Aspiration prior to laryngeal closure may be due to delayed triggering of the swallow.

_____ Aspiration prior to laryngeal closure may be due to impaired linguapalatal valving.

_____ Aspiration prior to laryngeal closure may be due to impaired laryngeal closure.

_____ Aspiration during maximum laryngeal closure is due to impaired laryngeal closure.

_____ Aspiration during maximum laryngeal closure is due to residue.

_____ Aspiration after or between swallows is due to residue falling into the airway once the larynx reopens.

_____ Aspiration after or between swallows is due to impaired laryngeal closure.

24. During the clinical evaluation of swallowing, all of the following would suggest risk of aspiration EXCEPT

a. a normal voice quality.

b. a breathy voice quality.

c. a history of vocal fold paralysis/paresis.

d. a gurgly or wet voice quality.

e. the sensation of food sticking in the throat after a swallow.

f. an ineffective and weak cough.

25. Aspiration during maximum laryngeal closure

a. warrants referral of the patient to an otolaryngologist with experience evaluating the larynx.

b. warrants a referral to a gastroenterologist to evaluate the pharyngoesophageal sphincter.

c. may be prevented or reduced using positional or swallowing maneuvers during swallowing.

d. Both (a) and (c) are correct, but not (b).

e. All of the above are correct.

f. None of the above are correct.

26. TRUE or FALSE (circle one): Observation of a pharyngoesophageal prominence (i.e., cricopharyngeal bar) during the swallow does not always mean that the opening is restricted and associated with hypopharyngeal residue.

27. TRUE or FALSE (circle one): The PES opening cannot be adequately tested if the patient cannot tolerate administration of a large liquid bolus (e.g., 20 cc).

28. TRUE or FALSE (circle one): The optimal method of determining whether the PES opening is adequate during the swallow is to obtain measures in the lateral plane only.

29. All of the following are true statements regarding videofluoroscopic observations at the level of the PES EXCEPT

    a. the timing of the PES opening should be determined in the context of the timing of other swallow gestures.

    b. the timing of the PES opening should be considered delayed based on bolus arrival in the hypopharynx.

    c. bolus contrast normally clears the walls of the PES completely upon completion of the swallow.

    d. the PES opening may be reduced related to absent or reduced hyolaryngeal elevation.

    e. the PES opening may have the appearance of a prominence due to thinning of the pharyngeal wall immediately above this region.

30. TRUE or FALSE (circle one): The esophageal screen at the end of a DSS is the same as an esophagram study.

31. An esophageal screen procedure is conducted in the LATERAL / A/P (circle one) plane while the patient STANDS UPRIGHT / SITS (circle one). The patient is administered a 5-mL / 20-mL (circle one) LIQUID / PASTE (circle one) bolus, or 15-mm barium. If the patient exhibits abnormal esophageal MOTILITY / STRUCTURAL ABNORMALITY (circle one), they will be referred for manometry testing, whereas observation of abnormal esophageal MOTILITY / STRUCTURAL ABNORMALITY (circle one) warrants referral for a transnasal esophagoscopy.

8

Dynamic Swallow Study: Objective Measures and Normative Data in Adults Questions

1. <u>TRUE</u> or <u>FALSE</u> (circle one): A team of dysphagia experts working together to calibrate subjective impressions through consensus can be expected to reliably make the same qualitative assessment (subjective judgment) of videofluoroscopic recordings related to hyolaryngeal excursion, pharyngeal constriction, and pharyngoesophageal segment (PES) opening during swallowing.

2. <u>TRUE</u> or <u>FALSE</u> (circle one): Transit time parameters previously defined by Dr. Logemann (1983) cannot be consistently performed on head and neck patients who have undergone resection of the structures typically used as landmarks.

3. <u>TRUE</u> or <u>FALSE</u> (circle one): A combined qualitative and quantitative approach, including measures of displacement and duration of gestures during deglutition, can be compared with normal measures by age group to improve the likelihood of accurately identifying someone with dysphagia and its characteristics for improved treatment planning.

4. Objective measures of videofluoroscopic recordings

   a. enable maintenance of meaningful measures to compare across individuals studied.

   b. enable comparison of pre- and posttreatment outcomes or progression over time.

   c. can elucidate qualitative impressions of bolus timing, flow, and clearance.

   d. provide a consistent method for characterizing the physiology underlying impaired deglutition.

   e. can be used to inform the best approach for intervention or habilitation/rehabilitation with a patient.

   f. All of the above.

5. Although not consistent with the experience of the authors, typical barriers reported by peers regarding the use of objective measurements to analyze videofluoroscopy recordings include

   a. the time spent completing measures is cost prohibitive.

   b. they do not change or contribute to diagnosis or treatment planning in a meaningful way.

   c. they are too difficult to replicate in the typical clinical setting.

   d. they do not help track pre- to posttreatment progress.

   e. All of the above statements are true.

   f. The only correct statements are (a) and (c).

6. <u>TRUE</u> or <u>FALSE</u> (circle one): The primary purpose in completing a videofluoroscopy evaluation is to determine the presence/absence of aspiration, making completion of measures unnecessary.

7. All of the following are reasons to complete a videofluoroscopic evaluation EXCEPT to

    a. identify the presence/absence of aspiration.

    b. determine the risk of aspiration in an individual, even if aspiration is not observed during the evaluation.

    c. determine the presence/absence of pneumonia.

    d. determine the presence/absence and characteristics of the patient's response if they are observed to aspirate.

    e. evaluate bolus flow, timing, and clearance related to bolus consistency as well as volume and stage of deglutition.

    f. determine the physiology associated with normal and abnormal aspects of deglutition.

    g. determine the patient's potential for intervention or treatment.

    h. monitor change or progression over time or relative to treatment.

8. TRUE or FALSE (circle one): There is a standardized method for conducting and evaluating videofluoroscopy evaluation of deglutition used by all speech-language pathologists in every state in the United States.

9. TRUE or FALSE (circle one): Consistent acquisition of objective measures of videofluoroscopic evaluations of deglutition has been shown to offer different measures indicative of aspiration pneumonia risk in particular patient populations.

10. All of the following are examples of bolus transit measures EXCEPT

    a. the initiation of anterior and superior movement of the hyoid bone.

    b. the time of the first movement of the bolus head past the posterior nasal spine as a zero point indicating the entry of the bolus into the pharynx.

    c. the time at which the bolus reaches the base of the vallecula to mark the end of oropharyngeal transit and the beginning of hypopharyngeal transit.

    d. the time at which the bolus head exits from the valleculae to mark the initiation of hypopharyngeal transit.

    e. the time at which the bolus head enters the upper esophageal sphincter (UES) as the sphincter opens.

    f. the time at which the tail of the bolus clears the PES marking the end of the pharyngeal bolus transit period.

    g. oropharyngeal transit time.

    h. oroduodenal transit time.

    i. hypopharyngeal transit time.

    j. total pharyngeal transit time.

    k. Both (a) and (h) are incorrect examples of bolus transit times.

    l. All of the above are correct examples of bolus transit times.

11. Results from comparison of bolus transit times in 62 subjects under age 65 years and 83 subjects over age 65 years, all of whom did not have dysphagia, showed

    a. prolonged transit times, in general, in the older age group.

    b. significantly prolonged transit times for 1-cc, 3-cc, and 20-cc bolus sizes in the elderly group compared with the younger group.

    c. a subgroup of 23 normal elderly subjects without medical conditions showed prolonged transit times compared with the younger group.

    d. All of the above.

12. TRUE or FALSE (circle one): Prolonged pharyngeal transit time is not typically associated with an increased risk for aspiration pneumonia.

13. Match the following times associated with swallow gestures and their correct operational definition.

    A. Airway closure

    B. Hyoid displacement

    C. PES opening

    D. PES closing

    E. Return of the epiglottis to rest position

    F. PES opening duration

    G. Duration of airway closure

    _____ The duration of time between approximation of the epiglottis against the arytenoid cartilage (AEclosure) and return of the epiglottis to preswallow position (Em)

    _____ The time at which the PES closes associated with the tail of the bolus fully in the esophagus; this gesture defines the end of the oropharyngeal swallow

    _____ The time at which airway closure occurs during the swallow is associated with onset of the initiation of elevation of the aryepiglottic folds (AEstart) and the time at which the downward folding of the epiglottis (AEclose) makes contact with the arytenoid cartilages

    _____ The duration of time between the first opening of the PES and PES closure

    _____ The time at which the PES appears to open associated with entry of the bolus head

    _____ The time at which the epiglottis appears to return to the preswallow position; this gestural time marks full restoration of an open respiratory status following a discrete swallow

    _____ The initiation of superior-anterior displacement of the hyoid bone (H1) associated with a swallow followed by the time at which the hyoid bone reaches its maximum superior-anterior excursion during the swallow (H2); the time at which the hyoid shows its first return movement to rest position (H3) also allows measurement of the total duration of time taken associated with hyoid displacement during the swallow

14. The time at which measurement of maximum hyoid bone displacement from baseline position is provided by

   a. H1.

   b. H2.

   c. H3.

   d. H4.

   e. Both (a) and (b).

15. The onset of the swallow response is considered to be provided at the time of this swallow gesture.

   a. The time at which the arytenoid cartilage makes contact with the aryepiglottic fold

   b. The time at which the bolus reaches the valleculae

   c. The time of the first movement of the hyoid bone in the anterior-superior direction

   d. The time at which the bolus head enters the pharyngoesophageal segment

16. Match the following temporal measures to their correct definition.

   A. Oropharyngeal transit time

   B. Hypopharyngeal transit time

   C. Total pharyngeal transit time

   D. PES opening duration

   E. Airway closure duration

   F. Hyoid maximum duration

   _____ The duration of time from PES opening to PES closing (Pcl–Pop)

   _____ The total time between the oropharyngeal and hypopharyngeal transit times (BP2–B1)

   _____ The duration of the bolus transit through the oropharynx as measured from the point in time when the bolus passes the posterior nasal spine (B1) to the time the bolus exits from the valleculae (BV2)

   _____ The duration of maximum hyoid displacement as measured from the point of maximum anterior-superior displacement during the swallow until the hyoid bone initiates a return to preswallow position (H3–H2)

   _____ The duration of supraglottic airway closure during the swallow indicated by the time from arytenoid cartilage approximation to the epiglottis until the epiglottis returns to preswallow position (Em–AEc)

   _____ The duration taken for the bolus to transit through the hypopharynx as measured from the time the bolus head initiates exit from the valleculae (BV2) to the time the bolus tail clears the PES (BP2)

17. <u>TRUE</u> or <u>FALSE</u> (circle one): The position of the UES is consistently located at the level of the PES associated with cervical vertebrae 5 to 6 in all individuals.

18. Label the following statements as either true (T) or false (F) regarding swallow gesture times.

    _____ As the size of the bolus increases, the duration of PES opening (Pcl–Pop) increases.

    _____ As bolus size increases, the duration of PES opening increases.

    _____ As bolus size increases, the total duration of oropharyngeal swallow also increases.

    _____ The duration of hyoid bone maximum displacement is longer during swallows of paste than for 3-cc liquid boluses.

    _____ The duration of PES opening is prolonged during swallows of a paste bolus than for liquid boluses.

    _____ The duration of airway closure (Em–AEclose) is longer during smaller bolus sizes than larger bolus sizes.

    _____ The duration of maximum hyoid bone displacement (H3–H2) is reduced in elderly individuals (>65 years) without dysphagia compared with younger normal individuals for 1-cc, 3-cc, and 20-cc liquid bolus sizes.

19. Identify all of the following relationships between bolus transit times and oropharyngeal swallow gestures that have been found to remain consistent between subjects and across bolus categories (consistencies and volumes).

    _____ Maximum pharyngeal constriction (PAmax) always occurs before maximal distension of the UES (PESmax).

    _____ Initiation of airway closure indicated by elevation of the aryepiglottic folds (AEstart) always begins prior to PES opening (Pop).

    _____ The bolus always arrives at the PES prior to its opening (Pop).

    _____ The PES always closes at the same time or just after the bolus tail clears the sphincter (BP2).

    _____ Onset of UES opening (Pop) always occurs before the time of maximum hyoid to larynx approximation (HLx).

20. Match the following spatial measures with their correct operational definition.

A. Maximum hyoid displacement

B. Referent hold position

C. Pharyngeal constriction ratio

D. Maximum opening of the PES

E. Maximum approximation of the larynx and hyoid

_____ The spatial measure defined as the referent position of deglutition structures while the individual holds a 1-cc bolus in the oral cavity

_____ The width at maximum distention of the PES during the swallow as a liquid bolus passes through

_____ The maximum anterior to superior change in hyoid bone position from referent hold position

_____ The distance between the larynx and hyoid bone during their maximum approximation during the swallow

_____ The ratio of pharyngeal area measured in the lateral view at the point of maximum constriction during the swallow divided by the pharyngeal area in the referent hold position

21. TRUE or FALSE (circle one): Displacement measures are typically made with reference to a "hold" position, which is defined as the position of the structures involved in deglutition while holding a 1-cc liquid bolus in the oral cavity prior to a swallow.

22. TRUE or FALSE (circle one): The optimal bolus for determining the true PESmax is the 1-cc liquid bolus.

23. Identify the correct timing sequence (1–15) of each of the following swallow gestures during the course of a swallow within Video 8–1, BTSGTiming on the Plural + Plus Companion Website.

_____ HLm: The timing of maximum approximation of the hyoid bone and larynx

_____ B1: The onset of supraglottic closure indicated by movement of the arytenoid cartilage elevation and downfolding of the epiglottis

_____ H1: The head of the bolus reaching the base of the valleculae

_____ BP2: The timing of the tail of the bolus clearing the PES

_____ PAm: The timing of maximum pharyngeal constriction

_____ BV1: The head of the bolus beginning to exit from the valleculae

_____ BP1: The timing of the hyoid bone at its maximum superior-anterior excursion during the swallow

_____ Pcl: The timing of the first closure of the PES closing on the tail of the bolus

_____ AEc: The time at which the PES appears open

_____ AEs: The first superior-anterior displacement of the hyoid that results in a swallow

_____ BV2: The epiglottis approximating the arytenoid cartilages indicating supraglottic closure

_____ Pop: The head of the bolus first enters the UES as it opens

_____ H2: The timing of the maximal opening of the PES

_____ ONSET: The first movement of the bolus past the posterior nasal spine

_____ PESm: The timing of maximal distension of the UES

24. Watch Video 8–2, YngEldSwallow on the Companion Website. The younger individual is shown on the left and the older individual is on the right. Based on your observation of this clip, select the following accurate comparisons of the two individual swallow recordings.

_____ The younger individual exhibited prolonged pharyngeal bolus transit time during the swallow.

_____ The older individual showed a delayed onset of the swallow compared with the younger individual.

_____ The older individual exhibited pharyngeal residue after the first swallow, whereas the younger individual did not exhibit pharyngeal residue.

_____ The younger individual exhibited two swallows to clear the entire bolus administered during the swallow trial.

_____ The older individual showed reduced pharyngeal constriction compared with the younger individual.

25. TRUE or FALSE (circle one): The referent hold position used to complete spatial measures of videofluoroscopy is analogous to a relaxed rest position of the upper airway structures that participate in deglutition.

26. Measurement of maximum hyoid displacement during the swallow

    a. can help explain reduced PES opening in some patients with dysphagia as the elevation of the hyoid and larynx contribute to this swallow gesture.

    b. is an important spatial measure reflective of velopharyngeal closure that results in nasal regurgitation when impaired or reduced.

    c. is associated with linguapalatal valving important to bolus containment in the oral cavity prior to initiation of bolus pharyngeal transit.

    d. is typically normal in individuals subsequent to floor-of-mouth or base-of-tongue resection or postradiation.

27. The distance between the hyoid bone and larynx during maximum approximation during the swallow

    a. is a measure used to demonstrate muscle tension dysphonia.

    b. is larger for liquid boluses than paste bolus consistency.

    c. is considered to reflect information relevant to airway protection and PES opening during the swallow.

    d. correlates with onset of linguapalatal opening as the bolus initiates transit through the pharynx.

28. TRUE or FALSE (circle one): The pharyngeal area measured during maximum constriction during the swallow (PAmax) has been found to be significantly different between males and females. In general, males exhibit a larger average PAmax than females.

29. The pharyngeal constriction ratio is

    a. a ratio of pharyngeal area during maximum pharyngeal constriction during the swallow to the pharyngeal area during quiet breathing in a relaxed position.

    b. larger in individuals older than 65 years compared with those younger than 65 years.

    c. considered normal when it surpasses 0.20 cm^2.

    d. a three-dimensional measurement.

30. TRUE or FALSE (circle one): Persistent pharyngeal residue associated with reduced pharyngeal constriction is associated with a smaller pharyngeal constriction ratio measure.

31. Label the following statements as either true (T) or false (F) regarding spatial swallowing measures.

    _____ PESmax has been shown to be reduced in elderly (>65 years) compared with younger (≤65 years) individuals.

    _____ The maximum displacement of the hyoid bone (Hmax) has been shown to be reduced in elderly (>65 years) compared with younger (≤65 years) individuals.

    _____ Bolus size has been found to affect measures of the distance between the hyoid bone and the larynx during maximum approximation during the swallow, with the larger distance associated with larger bolus sizes.

    _____ The maximum opening of the pharyngoesophageal segment (PESmax) has been found to increase with increased bolus size.

    _____ Increased bolus sizes have been associated with increased displacement of the hyoid bone at its maximum displacement (Hmax).

32. Select all of the following findings that are true resulting from studies of patterns between spatial and gesture measures during videofluoroscopy as described in the textbook.

   _____ An association was found between impaired PES function and pharyngeal dilation and weakness as indicated by increased measures of pharyngeal area during the referent hold position (PAhold) associated with decreased opening of the PES (PESmax).

   _____ Investigation of pharyngeal changes after cricopharyngeal myotomy for treatment of PES obstruction found that PESmax increased during swallowing of a 20-cc liquid bolus and pharyngeal constriction ratio (PCR) decreased, suggesting improved outcomes.

   _____ PCR studied in individuals with myotonic muscular dystrophy was shown to be normal or reduced compared with normal individuals.

   _____ PCR has been shown to indicate the risk factor for aspiration with values under 0.20 cm², indicative of persons who were three times more likely to aspirate compared with those with a value greater than 0.32 cm² who did not aspirate.

   _____ PCR has been shown to inversely covary with pharyngeal manometry pressure measures such that smaller constriction ratios were associated with higher manometry pressure measures during swallowing. In addition, normal PCR values were associated with normal manometry pressure values, whereas abnormal PCR values reflective of impaired pharyngeal constriction were associated with abnormally reduced manometry pressure values.

   _____ Measures of PCR and pharyngeal area during referent hold position demonstrated that elderly individuals (>65 years) demonstrate significantly larger areas than younger individuals (≤65 years) and a greater distance between the hyoid and larynx during referent hold, suggesting that the pharynx is longer in elderly than in younger individuals as well.

33. All of the following are advantages to completed standardized objective measures of videofluoroscopic evaluation of deglutition EXCEPT that it

   a. permits a comparison between normal and abnormal data for improved diagnostic precision in identifying the presence/absence of dysphagia.

   b. provides a means for characterizing unique patient populations.

   c. does not allow us to expand interpretation to biomechanical deviations but can allow us to identify the presence or absence of aspiration.

   d. allows comparison between other instrumental measures of swallow function (e.g., electromyography or manometry).

34. The bolus clearance ratio (BCR) of .60 that was obtained during Video 8–3, BCR on the Companion Website indicates

    a. the proportion of the total bolus entering the pharynx that was cleared during the swallow.

    b. the proportion of the total bolus entering the pharynx remaining after the swallow.

    c. the maximum pharyngeal constriction area.

    d. the maximum pharyngeal area that the bolus residue occupied.

35. All of the following statements are true regarding the displacement and duration measures for the patient example displayed in the textbook Figure 8–2 EXCEPT

    a. Hyolaryngeal excursion was reduced compared with normative measures.

    b. The pharyngeal constrictor ratio (PCR) was larger than normative measures, indicating reduced pharyngeal constriction during the swallow.

    c. The maximum opening of the PES was greater than the normative measure values.

    d. Total pharyngeal transit time was prolonged compared with normative measures.

9

Other Technologies in Dysphagia Assessment Questions

1. A comprehensive dysphagia evaluation should include assessment of the _____ . Approximately _____ of individuals who localize the site of the dysphagia above the _____ have an _____ etiology for their symptom.

2. Transnasal esophagoscopy (TNE):

   a. can be used as a first-line tool to diagnose esophageal pathology in those with pill or solid food dysphagia complaints.

   b. has been shown to be unsafe as an in-office procedure due to the use of sedation.

   c. is precluded for use in the head and neck cancer population.

   d. is not typically considered a tool for use in evaluating individuals with dysphagia.

3. The _____ in the esophagus, or GOOSE, is the esophageal counterpart to the _____. This exam is completed after the FEES evaluation after it is determined that no _____ or _____ abnormality is responsible for the patient's dysphagia and a comorbid _____ disorder is suspected. During the GOOSE, the endoscope is passed through the upper _____ sphincter into the cervical _____ during a saliva or water swallow. During administration of bolus swallows, the GOOSE procedure enables observation of _____ peristalsis during swallowing. At the end of the GOOSE, a retroflexed view of the _____ is obtained from within the stomach.

4. Ultrasound:

   a. can be used to observe the entire oropharyngeal swallow and diagnose aspiration.

   b. is prohibitively expensive to use clinically.

   c. is best used to study the hard bony and cartilaginous framework involved in swallowing.

   d. is a radiation-free option to the DSS for evaluation of some aspects of deglutition.

5. Scintigraphy:

   a. enables views of radio tracer materials during a DSS.

   b. is unsafe for use in pediatric populations due to the excessive exposure to radiation.

   c. can be used to measure the quantity and location of a nuclear tracer, Tc-99mm, to identify aspiration.

   d. is currently being used in most clinical settings to study swallowing physiology.

6. Select all of the following items that correctly identify roles for magnetic resonance imaging (MRI) and high-resolution computed tomography (CT) applied to dysphagia.

_____ Functional MRI enables investigation of neural pathways associated with deglutition activities.

_____ MRI can be used to study deglutition in the upright position in the same way a DSS is conducted.

_____ CT can be used to provide three-dimensional (3D) reconstruction of the aerodigestive tract anatomy and its function during swallowing.

_____ Dynamic MRI enables high-resolution study of the anatomic structures involved in deglutition.

_____ Functional MRI is currently being used to stimulate impaired neural pathways to facilitate improved swallowing function.

_____ CT enables image acquisition with a cost-efficient and low-dose radiation option to the DSS.

7. Pharyngeal and esophageal manometry provides distinction between all of the following EXCEPT

a. velopharyngeal closure.

b. pharyngeal weakness.

c. poor pharyngeal/cricopharyngeal coordination.

d. incomplete upper esophageal sphincter relaxation.

8. High-resolution manometry (HRM) has largely replaced conventional _____.

HRM is performed with a 2.7- to 4.2-mm diameter catheter containing _____

circumferential solid state sensors with _____ cm spacing. Conventional manometry

catheters contained only _____ sensors spaced widely apart. HRM provides a unique high-

fidelity measurement of _____, _____, and _____

physiology during swallowing.

9. All of the following are accurate statements about multichannel intraluminal impedance EXCEPT

    a. when combined with pH testing, acid and non-acid reflux can be quantified.

    b. impedance testing measures resistance to current flow. Given the high ionic concentration of food and refluxate materials, the impedance signal will drop because resistance to current flow drops.

    c. this method cannot be combined with manometry.

    d. All of the above are accurate statements.

10. The SmartPill®:

    a. measures the pressures and rate of movement of the bolus during oropharyngeal swallows.

    b. transmits information about transit of a bolus through the stomach, small bowel, and colon.

    c. enables measures of gastric and colonic transit times of meals consumed during a study.

    d. can only be used during consumption of barium radio-opaque contrast materials.

    e. All of the above responses are correct.

    f. Responses (b) and (c) are correct.

11. Ambulatory pH testing of gastroesophageal reflux disease (GERD):

    a. entails the use of a distal sensor placed above the lower esophageal sphincter or gastroesophageal junction to measure reflux episodes.

    b. can be conducted using a sensor that is hardwired to a catheter or using a wireless telemetry capsule.

    c. can be diagnosed by placement of a pH sensor in the hypopharynx.

    d. can be determined during dual probe pH testing.

    e. All of the above responses are correct EXCEPT for (c).

    f. None of the above responses are correct.

12. TRUE or FALSE (circle one): The same method of wireless pH probe testing used to diagnose gastroesophageal reflux disease can be used to diagnose laryngopharyngeal reflux.

10

The Treatment Plan: Behavioral Approaches Questions

1. The treatment plan for an individual with dysphagia should consider relevant information from

   a. the patient's medical history/chart review.

   b. current physical examinations or clinical evaluations, including cognitive status.

   c. findings on the bedside or clinical evaluation of swallowing.

   d. results of the videofluoroscopic study.

   e. related examinations or studies such as esophagram, manometry, endoscopy, and so forth.

   f. the patient's current setting, available resources, and support network.

   g. All of the above.

2. TRUE or FALSE (circle one): It is rarely the case that a treatment plan will incorporate a recommendation for a referral or additional tests before a final decision and plan is formulated.

3. Concerns arising regarding laryngeal function pertinent to safe swallowing require a referral or further evaluation by

   a. a neurologist.

   b. a pulmonologist.

   c. an otolaryngologist.

   d. a radiologist.

   e. an occupational therapist.

   f. None of the above.

   g. All of the above.

4. Concerns about dental or oral hygiene status affecting deglutition require referral or further evaluation by

   a. a dentist.

   b. a prosthodontist.

   c. a dental hygienist.

   d. an oral surgeon.

   e. an otolaryngologist.

   f. Any of the above, depending on the patient.

   g. None of the above.

5. TRUE or FALSE (circle one): Once the evaluation of deglutition is completed, the final treatment plan and recommendations should incorporate a consideration of the referring professional's concerns and questions as well as the patient's questions or complaints.

6. The treatment options may be classified as all of the following EXCEPT

    a. behavioral.

    b. medical.

    c. surgical.

    d. astrological.

    e. All of the above are correct classifications.

    f. None of the above are correct classifications.

7. The following professionals all may provide behavioral treatment to patients diagnosed with dysphagia EXCEPT

    a. a primary care physician.

    b. a speech-language pathologist.

    c. an occupational therapist.

    d. a physical therapist.

    e. a nurse.

    f. a dietitian.

    g. All of the above provide behavioral intervention.

8. TRUE or FALSE (circle one): In most cases, knowing the primary etiology of dysphagia is enough information to plan treatment for the patient.

9. Behavioral management/treatment of dysphagia is used when

    a. strength, endurance, and/or mobility of structures involved in swallowing are intact.

    b. swallowing was shown to appear safer through the use of postural compensation methods.

    c. swallowing was shown to appear worsened through the use of a facilitative device or facilitative maneuver.

    d. swallowing delay or initiation is unresponsive to sensory stimuli such as mechanical or thermal sensory applications.

    e. All of the above are correct.

    f. None of the above are correct.

10. *Identify which of the following statements offers the INCORRECT completion of this statement*: "Behavioral management focused on improving strength, mobility, and endurance of structures involved in deglutition _____."

   a. may improve pharyngoesophageal opening through strengthening of hyolaryngeal elevation musculature, such as the "Shaker exercises" that require sets of head elevation from a supine position such that the patient can see her/his toes upon raising.

   b. may improve lingual strength for propelling the bolus through the oropharynx through progressive resistance against a tongue pressure bulb placed orally requiring applied lingual pressure at a proportion of maximum force capability for a training effect.

   c. may improve tongue–pharynx contact through resistance of tongue retraction during swallowing via holding the anterior tongue between the teeth (i.e., Masako maneuver).

   d. includes progressive resistance exercises directed toward expiratory musculature to improve respiratory expiration needed for an effective cough.

   e. can improve esophageal motility by providing electrical stimulation to the superficial musculature of the anterior neck.

11. Behavioral management is indicated for all of the following impairments EXCEPT

   a. weakness or limited movement of the moving structures such as the lips, mandible, tongue, pharynx, larynx, or pharyngoesophageal segment.

   b. failure to protect the airway related to reduced or absent hyolaryngeal elevation or impaired laryngeal seal/closure.

   c. severe mucositis and fibrosis during a course of chemoradiation treatment for head and neck cancer.

   d. poor oral control of food boluses due to weakened strength, endurance, and mobility of the tongue subsequent to head and neck surgery or poststroke.

   e. weak or absent pharyngeal constrictor function associated with advanced stage amyotrophic lateral sclerosis.

   f. Only (c) and (e) would be examples where behavioral management is considered inappropriate.

   g. All of the above are appropriate for behavioral management.

   h. None of the above are appropriate for behavioral management.

12. The expiratory muscle strength training program developed by Sapienza and Wheeler (2006) has been shown to

    a. benefit only respiratory function and improve cough function in patients diagnosed with Parkinson disease.

    b. improve airway safety and swallow-related behaviors such as hyolaryngeal excursion during swallowing.

    c. be associated with worsened airway protection as evidenced by worsened scores on the Penetration-Aspiration Scale.

    d. None of the above.

    e. All of the above.

13. Lee Silverman Voice Therapy

    a. focuses on improving vocal loudness in individuals with Parkinson disease.

    b. recalibrates individuals with Parkinson disease to increase effort levels during speaking to improve intelligibility and voice production.

    c. is associated with reduced oral and pharyngeal transit times as well as reduced pharyngeal residue posttreatment.

    d. is associated with improved bolus formation posttreatment.

    e. All of the above.

    f. Only (a) and (b) are true.

14. TRUE or FALSE (circle one): Behavioral management approaches for treating dysphagia are mainly determined based on the principles of strength, mobility, and endurance without scientific evidence to support their use.

15. TRUE or FALSE (circle one): As with speech therapy approaches, the use of non-swallowing-related strength and mobility exercises has not been shown to benefit swallowing function.

16. Application of behavioral treatment regimens should consider all of the following EXCEPT

    a. uniform and consistent use of the treatment protocol with all impaired individuals regardless of their diagnosis or current function level because these programs should work with everyone.

    b. the specific instructions and methods demonstrated in the literature as effective.

    c. the dosage required for clinical gains, with dosage defined by the number of exercise repetitions per day and the number of days per week for a prescribed duration to achieve clinical gains.

    d. the manner and frequency of knowledge of results necessary for the patient to independently carry out accurate practice outside of the therapy room.

    e. pre- and posttreatment indicators/measures reflective of clinical gains expected from the treatment method.

17. TRUE or FALSE (circle one): Exercise programs to improve oral, pharyngeal, and laryngeal structure strength, mobility, endurance, and agility require head/neck and upper body postural stability (i.e., stable platform) against which the target structure can move. If this is not in place, consultation with occupational therapy and physical therapy may be indicated to supplement or set the stage for such treatment intervention.

18. Biofeedback or performance feedback methods that may help improve deglutition in the face of impaired sensory mechanisms or sensorimotor function include

    a. flexible nasoendoscopy for direct imaging of pharyngeal structures.

    b. electromyography for feedback of esophageal pressure.

    c. manometry to provide electrical information about individual muscle fiber motor units or groups of muscles activating during contraction associated with deglutition functions.

    d. use of the intra-oral pressure transducer (IOPI), which provides audio sounds associated with the sounds of the swallow to enhance the patient's coordination and timing of the swallow.

19. Patient adherence to any treatment program can be hampered by all of the following EXCEPT

    a. lack of understanding of the treatment rationale.

    b. information overload regarding the treatment and its implementation.

    c. forgetfulness.

    d. high motivation to avoid long-term feeding tube use.

20. Coordination of respiration and swallowing can be trained to improve airway protection and clearance by

    a. using biofeedback to show respiratory nasal airflow activity relative to swallowing.

    b. asking patients to hawk and then spit out their secretions.

    c. training patients to swallow during the midexpiratory phase of breathing and then continue exhalation upon completion of the swallow.

    d. All of the above are correct responses.

    e. Responses (a) and (c) are both correct.

21. Surface electrode neuromuscular electrical stimulation of swallowing

    a. applies thermostimulation and ultrasound to external musculature of the throat important to hyolaryngeal elevation.

    b. requires an intact lower motor unit to stimulate activation of the neuromuscular unit to enhance tone and strength in weakened muscles involved in swallowing.

    c. is used to stimulate functional activation of musculature involved in swallowing to enhance the timely onset and sequential contraction of pharyngeal musculature via surface muscular stimulation.

    d. has definitively been proven to cure dysphagia and can be used with everyone demonstrating severe impairment of swallowing function.

    e. administers electrical stimulation directly to the motor neuron to target musculature.

22. Direct muscle stimulation

    a. requires an electrode placed directly into the target muscle.

    b. has been shown to result in improved airway production when systematically applied over several months in an animal model.

    c. utilizes cortical stimulation resulting in coordinated patterns of activation of peripheral swallowing musculature.

    d. can be implemented readily in the clinic by a speech-language pathologist.

    e. Both (a) and (b) are correct.

    f. All of the above are correct.

    g. None of the above.

23. TRUE or FALSE (circle one): A study by Langmore and colleagues (2016) showed that the inclusion of transcutaneous electrical stimulation during the swallowing exercise protocol in those with head and neck cancer was beneficial.

24. Explain how functional electrical stimulation (FES) is distinct from neuromuscular electrical stimulation (NMES) treatment methods.

25. Identify all of the following examples of dysphagia treatment methods that utilize bolus manipulation.

    _____ Modify the size of bolus eaten (small bites versus large volume)

    _____ Ask the patient to flex her/his neck during a swallow

    _____ Placing the bolus on the posterior left tongue, which appears stronger than the anterior tongue

    _____ Modify bolus viscosity (liquid versus paste)

    _____ Instruct the patient on progressive strengthening of her/his tongue over 16 weeks using the IOPI

    _____ Use of chemosensory stimulants such as sour or sweet

    _____ Modify the temperature of the bolus (cold versus hot)

    _____ Instruct the patient to swallow hard during each swallow

    _____ Air pulses applied to the oral cavity and oropharyngeal mucosa

26. Modifications of bolus viscosity
    a. should always be done when aspiration is observed in a patient.
    b. must consider the Newtonian characteristics of the bolus being modified.
    c. include thickening liquids with starch or gum-based materials, which both result in the same range of viscosity impact on liquids.
    d. can be done using the same thickening methods on all liquids.
    e. are well defined and studied, resulting in standard implementation across clinic settings.
    f. All of the above.
    g. None of the above.

27. Identify all of the following treatment approaches for dysphagia that utilize postural compensations.

_____ Tilting the body laterally or posteriorly to divert the bolus away from the airway or toward musculature that appears intact and functional

_____ Anterior head flexion during each swallow to prevent aspiration before or during the swallow

_____ Encouraging throat clearing or coughing after each swallow is completed

_____ Limiting the patient to drinking nectar or honey-thick liquids

_____ Providing jaw support to an infant for improved management of drinking through a nipple

_____ Repeated head lifting from a supine position to strengthen the anterior hyolaryngeal musculature

_____ Rotating the head toward the side of impaired pharyngeal or laryngeal musculature to compress that side and encourage flow of the bolus through the functional or stronger side

_____ Recommendation of tube feedings

28. Match the following facilitative maneuvers of dysphagia treatment with their correct definition or description.

    A. Effortful swallow

    B. Supraglottic swallow

    C. Super supraglottic swallow

    D. Mendelsohn maneuver

    E. Mandibular advancement

    _____ This approach is used to increase displacement and duration of hyoid and laryngeal movement during the swallow to prolong PES opening. The patient is instructed to swallow and hold while the hyoid and larynx are raised and to relax after a prolonged duration after the swallow has completed (e.g., up to 1–5 s or so).

    _____ Typically used with patients with airway closure timing delays or incomplete laryngeal closure during swallowing. The patient is instructed to put the bolus in the mouth and breath hold while swallowing and release the breath after the swallow is complete.

    _____ This method has been shown to be effective in patients with limited PES opening but with good control of oral structures such that they jut the jaw forward at the time of the swallow initiation.

    _____ Used typically in patients with weak pharyngeal constriction; patients are instructed to swallow as hard as they can and squeeze their swallow muscles harder.

    _____ Typically used with patients with airway closure timing issues or incomplete laryngeal closure during swallowing. The patient is instructed to bear down with great effort during swallowing to elicit supraglottic constriction for airway protection followed by an audible exhalation after the swallow is completed.

29. All of the following are examples of using facilitative devices to treat patients with feeding or swallowing problems EXCEPT

    a. modification of nipple flow/resistance or stiffness.

    b. administration of a bolus using a catheter and syringe.

    c. instructing the patient to swallow hard and squeeze her/his throat muscles.

    d. use of a palatal prosthesis to reshape the oral cavity, lower the hard palate, elevate the soft palate, or obturate the velopharyngeal port.

    e. All of the above are examples of using facilitative devices to treat dysphagia.

30. Identify all of the following treatment approaches for dysphagia that utilize selective stimulation to improve swallow initiation and timing.

_____ Reduce noise, light, and other distractions to enable orientation and focus on eating

_____ Provide verbal cues (e.g., say his/her name or cue a behavior) or visual cues to the patient (hold up a card, gesture to the patient, etc.)

_____ Use of a syringe and catheter to administer the bolus

_____ Stimulating the oral gums to provide mechanical stimulation to alert or orient oral structures during eating

_____ Repeated head lifting from a supine position to strengthen the anterior hyolaryngeal musculature

_____ Application of mechanical or vibratory stimulation to the faucial pillars to lower the mechanosensory threshold to stimulate onset of the swallow

_____ Ask the patient to flex his/her head anteriorly during a swallow to protect the airway

_____ Application of thermal stimulation via an icy laryngeal mirror to the anterior faucial pillars to improve swallow initiation

_____ Transcranial magnetic stimulation to trigger pharyngeal constriction during swallowing

31. The use of computer applications have been developed to

   a. aid in ensuring patient access to therapeutic instructions to help improve accurate practice at home.

   b. aid in patient adherence to prescribed therapeutic regimens.

   c. replace the role of clinicians involved in administering behavioral treatment.

   d. allow patients to self-diagnose and select their preferred treatment modality for practice.

   e. Both (a) and (b) are correct.

   f. Both (c) and (d) are correct.

   g. None of the above.

   h. All of the above.

32. Label the following statements as either true (T) or false (F) regarding dysphagia treatment.

_____ It is important that members of the dysphagia team meet with and communicate the final treatment plan to the patient and her/his caregivers and respond to all related questions about the plan.

_____ Pretreatment measures regarding the patient's swallowing quality of life and videofluoroscopic study can be compared with posttreatment studies and scores to determine progress or treatment outcome.

_____ Differing opinions among team members regarding patient treatment methods or plans should not be documented.

_____ The summary of findings for a patient with dysphagia should also include conclusions that the referring professional may not be able to independently determine, such as the etiology and severity of the impairment and its impact on nutrition and respiratory health and prognosis for improvement.

_____ It is only important that the treatment plan be disseminated to the caregivers in the patient's immediate environment.

_____ It may be important to post the treatment plan at the patient's bedside and include it in a hospital discharge plan.

_____ Recommendations for follow-up, if any, should be included in the report even though it is the responsibility of the patient's referring physician to monitor the patient and determine the need for follow-up visits or reevaluation.

_____ If a team sees a large number of patients, it is acceptable to allow time constraints to influence reduced priority of a thorough evaluation and critical review of each individual patient's situation in favor of improving efficiency.

33. TRUE or FALSE (circle one): Biomechanical timing and displacement measures from videofluoroscopy can be recorded across patients and time to allow evaluation of general treatment outcomes or characteristics of patient populations once enough patient evaluations and treatment outcomes have been recorded.

34. TRUE or FALSE (circle one): Biomechanical timing and displacement measures are not useful for documenting treatment outcomes.

35. TRUE or FALSE (circle one): A combination of qualitative assessments (e.g., presence/absence of aspiration) and biomechanical timing and displacement measures offers a thorough approach for evaluating videofluoroscopic evaluation of deglutition.

36. Determining treatment outcomes may include all of the following approaches EXCEPT

    a. consistent recording of pre- and posttreatment biomechanical measures.

    b. pre- and posttreatment completion of self-assessment tools reflecting functional eating.

    c. pre- and posttreatment laboratory studies reflective of nutritional and hydration levels.

    d. pre- and posttreatment imaging studies to reflect changes in pulmonary or other health status.

    e. sending the patient to a different facility where her/his treatment will be carried out and evaluated posttreatment.

37. <u>TRUE</u> or <u>FALSE</u> (circle one): Dysphagia is a disorder that does not require multiple professionals from different disciplines involved in the evaluation and treatment process

11

The Treatment Plan: Medical and Surgical Questions

1. <u>TRUE</u> or <u>FALSE</u> (circle one): Many medications are known to impact swallowing function such that identification of a prescription drug or combination thereof as the source of an individual's dysphagia would require a medical decision regarding pharmaceutical modification to help lessen or improve symptoms.

2. All of the following are true of individuals diagnosed with gastroesophageal reflux as the source of their dysphagia EXCEPT that they

    a. benefit most from behavioral intervention using progressive lingual strengthening exercises or the Shaker exercises.

    b. benefit most from medical or surgical management to reduce or eliminate damage to esophageal and pharyngeal tissues resulting from chronic acid and pepsin exposure.

    c. benefit from behavioral intervention utilizing lifestyle changes such as dietary modifications, eating more than 3 hr before going to bed, elevating the head of the bed by 4 to 6 in., and avoiding acidic or spicy foods.

    d. may be prescribed H2 blockers or proton-pump inhibitors by a physician.

    e. All of the above.

    f. None of the above.

3. Xerostomia

    a. involves excessive production of saliva.

    b. results in difficulty lubricating nonliquid boluses for effective swallowing clearance.

    c. never causes changes in the flora and fauna of the oral and pharyngeal cavities.

    d. never improves with increased hydration and oral hygiene.

    e. reduces in severity when eating spicy or acidic foods to stimulate salivation.

    f. All of the above.

4. All of the following individuals are examples of candidates for surgical management of dysphagia EXCEPT

   a. an infant with a cleft palate and lip.

   b. a patient subsequent to an oropharyngeal cancer surgical resection.

   c. a patient with a pharyngeal web that obstructs bolus flow and clearance.

   d. a patient with severe unilateral vocal fold paralysis resulting in impaired airway protection during the swallow.

   e. a patient with cricopharyngeal achalasia causing significant obstruction to bolus entry into the esophagus.

   f. a patient exhibiting a cricopharyngeal bar and thinning of the posterior pharyngeal wall as well as an enlarged pharynx during quiet breathing.

   g. a patient exhibiting a Zenker's diverticulum (out-pouching of the pharyngeal mucosa above the cricopharyngeus muscle and between the inferior pharyngeal constrictor fibers).

5. Achalasia occurs commonly among those with neuromuscular disease which is

   a. characterized by cricopharyngeal hypotonia.

   b. characterized by cricothyroid hyperfunction.

   c. characterized by cricopharyngeal hyperfunction.

   d. optimally treated with anticholinergic medications.

   e. optimally treated with proton-pump inhibitors (PPIs).

   f. None of the above are correct responses.

6. <u>TRUE</u> or <u>FALSE</u> (circle one): A majority of individuals with gastroesophageal reflux disease (GERD) report oropharyngeal dysphagia symptoms and exhibit a normal esophageal screen during their videofluoroscopic evaluation.

7. Use of proton-pump inhibitors for treatment of gastroesophageal reflux disease (GERD)

   a. requires consistent daily use for 2 to 3 months for optimal management of reflux symptoms.

   b. can be used intermittently whenever reflux symptoms flare.

   c. requires consistent daily use for more than 6 months until reflux symptoms are cured.

   d. is a preferred approach for treating chronic GERD prior to implementing a behavioral antireflux regimen.

   e. None of the above are correct responses.

   f. All of the above are correct responses.

8. Surgical treatment of achalasia could be achieved by

   a. endoscopic myotomy of the cricopharyngeal muscle.

   b. dilation using a catheter with an inflatable balloon placed through the upper esophageal sphincter (UES).

   c. adherence to a daily routine of proton-pump inhibitors for 2 to 3 months.

   d. implementation of reflux lifestyle modifications.

   e. Only (a) and (b) are correct responses.

   f. All of the above are correct responses.

9. Identify all of the following considered to be forms of medical therapy that could be used to treat dysphagia, depending upon the primary etiology and clinical features.

   _____ Expiratory muscle strength training

   _____ Proton-pump inhibitors (PPIs; e.g., omeprazole, pantoprazole, etc.)

   _____ H2 blocker medications (e.g., famotidine, ranitidine, etc.)

   _____ Shaker head-lift exercise

   _____ Endoscopic esophageal dilation

   _____ Transcutaneous neuromuscular electrical stimulation

   _____ Cricopharyngeal myotomy

   _____ Progressive lingual strength training

10. All of the following are strategies used to manage xerostomia EXCEPT

    a. minimize use of medications with a side effect of mucosal dryness.

    b. maximize oral hygiene to control bacterial growth.

    c. increase hydration and eating "wet" foods.

    d. increase the frequency of eating acidic and "pepper-hot" foods.

    e. prescription of pilocarpine medication.

    f. All of the above are strategies that reduce problems due to xerostomia.

    g. None of the above are correct strategies.

11. TRUE or FALSE (circle one): Individuals diagnosed with vocal fold paralysis have been shown to exhibit increased aspiration risk due to impaired laryngeal valving requiring surgical medialization of the vocal folds as a consistently effective treatment.

12. Cricopharyngeal achalasia can result from

    a. cricopharyngeal fibrosis subsequent to radiation treatment.

    b. inclusion body myositis.

    c. gastroesophageal reflux disease (GERD).

    d. iatrogenic scarring of the cricopharyngeus.

    e. stroke.

    f. None of the above are correct causes of achalasia.

    g. All of the above are correct causes of achalasia.

13. Upper esophageal sphincter opening during the pharyngeal swallow occurs due to all of the following EXCEPT

    a. anterosuperior displacement of the hyolaryngeal complex during swallowing.

    b. cricopharyngeal muscle relaxation.

    c. cricopharyngeal muscle contraction.

    d. positive pharyngeal constriction pressure propelling the bolus through the UES.

14. Match all of the following with their associated medical therapy approach.

    A. Microstomia (contracture of the oral commissure) due to scleroderma

    B. Nasal regurgitation due to severe velopharyngeal insufficiency in a child with cleft palate

    C. Fibrosis of the cricopharyngeus resulting in impaired upper esophageal sphincter opening during the pharyngeal swallow

    D. Esophageal stricture

    E. Not a medical therapy approach

    _____ Therabite jaw motion rehabilitation

    _____ Cricopharyngeal myotomy

    _____ Botox treatment administered to the orbicularis oris musculature

    _____ Endoscopic balloon dilation

    _____ Prosthetic palatal lift

    _____ Velopharyngeal flap surgery

12

Airway Considerations in Dysphagia Questions

1. Check all of the following that describe pharyngeal physiology contributing to airway protection during the pharyngeal phase of swallowing.

   _____ Anterosuperior positioning of the hyolaryngeal complex under the base of tongue

   _____ Velopharyngeal port closure

   _____ Approximation of the true vocal folds, false vocal folds, and aryepiglottic folds

   _____ Relaxation of the cricopharyngeal muscle

   _____ Sequential constriction of the constrictor muscles

   _____ Expiration preceding and following the swallow

2. Select all of the following considered to be pulmonary risk factors for aspiration pneumonia in those with dysphagia.

   _____ Open heart surgery

   _____ Diabetic coma

   _____ Weight gain

   _____ Base-of-tongue cancer and surgery

   _____ Loss of 10 lb during the past month

   _____ Eats meals in an upright position more than 2 hr before lying down in a distraction-free environment in the presence of caregivers

   _____ Aerobic instructor

   _____ Trach or ventilation tube in place

   _____ Myopic vision

   _____ Poor oral hygiene

   _____ Chronic obstructive pulmonary disease

   _____ Systemic inflammatory response syndrome

   _____ Lung cancer

3. Define and describe chest and cervical auscultation.

    _____

    _____

4. Select the following items that are examples of aspiration precautions for a patient on an oral diet.

    _____ Observe for struggle during eating, coughing, choking, and throat clearing

    _____ Minimize distractions by maintaining a quiet environment and not talking during meals

    _____ Monitor for tube migration before administering a feeding

    _____ Do not leave the patient unattended or unobserved during meals

    _____ Coordinate diet recommendations and restrictions with the physician's order for amount, frequency, and consistencies

    _____ Oral care and hygiene before and after meals

    _____ Check for residuals before feeding

    _____ Implementation of reflux precautions

    _____ Position the patient at 90° in a chair, if possible, to maintain a safe upper body position

    _____ Assess pulmonary status for clinical signs of aspiration

5. TRUE or FALSE (circle one): Individuals primarily receiving nutrition through a feeding tube (NG, NJ, GT/J) are not likely to experience aspiration from gastroesophageal reflux.

6. A strong indication of reflux and possibly aspiration is _____ following a feeding (especially a bolus feeding), with a full stomach.

7. TRUE or FALSE (circle one): An inflated endotracheal tube cuff ensures that exhaled air passes directly through the vocal folds to produce phonation.

8. TRUE or FALSE (circle one): Placement of a tracheostomy tube is associated with increased hyolaryngeal anterosuperior excursion during the pharyngeal stage of swallowing.

9. <u>TRUE</u> or <u>FALSE</u> (circle one): Glucose monitoring of pulmonary secretions is a reliable indicator of reflux into the airway.

10. <u>TRUE</u> or <u>FALSE</u> (circle one): The presence of food (or enteral feeding in the case of a tube-fed patient) in a tracheostomy or in endotracheal secretions indicates occurrence of an aspiration event that requires an immediate response from the treatment team.

11. <u>TRUE</u> or <u>FALSE</u> (circle one): A cuffed tracheostomy tube prevents aspiration from occurring, making it rare for someone using one to get pneumonia.

12. <u>TRUE</u> or <u>FALSE</u> (circle one): An individual using a positive pressure ventilator is capable of breathing independently.

13. Identify the type of tracheostomy tube displayed in Figure 12–1 (using A–C).

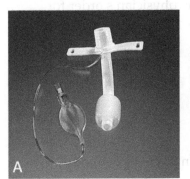 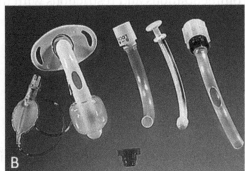 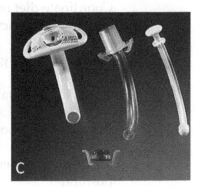

Figure 12-1. © 2023 Medtronic. All rights reserved. Used with the permission of Medtronic.

_____ Cuffed tracheostomy tube

_____ Uncuffed/cuffless tracheostomy tube

_____ Fenestrated tracheostomy tube

14. Define the following different types of tracheostomy tubes and the typical reason they are used.

a. Cuffed tracheostomy tube:

_____

_____

_____

b. Uncuffed/cuffless tracheostomy tube:

_____

_____

_____

c. Fenestrated tracheostomy tube:

_____

_____

_____

15. Identify possible negative consequences of tracheostomy tube placement on the pharyngeal swallow and respiratory protection.

_____

_____

_____

_____

_____

_____

13

Nutritional Considerations in Dysphagia Questions

1. <u>TRUE</u> or <u>FALSE</u> (circle one): Successful management of the nutritional and dietary needs of an individual with dysphagia only requires contributions from the medical team.

2. The responsibility of the dietitian is to (select all that apply)

    _____ assess the patient's hydration needs.

    _____ evaluate videofluoroscopic recordings of deglutition.

    _____ prescribe medications to reduce or eliminate reflux.

    _____ assess the patient's nutrition needs.

    _____ translate restrictions recommended by the dysphagia specialists into a diet.

    _____ refer the patient for surgical treatment.

    _____ contribute to transitions in dietary recommendations as needs change.

    _____ consider ways to make the prescribed diet palatable and appealing to the patient.

    _____ recommend modifications to tube feeding regimens for improved tolerance.

3. Nutritional assessment by a dietitian should be considered when a patient's means of _____ has been altered, when a change is _____, or when there are concerns about the _____ and/or _____ or _____ value of a patient's diet.

4. Characteristics of patients with dysphagia may determine
    a. their dietary needs.
    b. eligibility for funding sources supportive of nutritional needs.
    c. anticipated progress or deterioration in dietary needs over time.
    d. All of the above.

5. Of the following, select the signs that require a comprehensive nutritional evaluation.

_____ Significant changes in a patient's weight trends and hydration

_____ Loss of more than 20% of an individual's usual weight

_____ Loss of less than 10% of an individual's usual weight

_____ Loss of 4 lb within 48 hr in a 100-lb person

_____ Rising blood urea nitrogen (BUN) level indicative of dehydration

_____ Weight gain of 10 lb over 6 months in a 100-lb person

6. TRUE or FALSE (circle one): Rapid weight loss without adequate protein intake may impact the immune system and undermine the individual's resistance to disease and infection.

7. Match the following terms with the best description of their meaning or application to the context of an individual with dysphagia.

A. Serum albumin value

B. Prealbumin

C. C-reactive protein

D. Serum sodium and blood urea nitrogen (BUN)

_____ A positive acute phase protein that is used as an indicator of stress or inflammation

_____ Referred to as a "negative acute phase protein" that is considered to be a sensitive indicator of current protein status; it should never be considered alone as it can be lowered by inflammation, infection, or metabolic stressors regardless of nutritional status

_____ Elevated values occur in individuals suffering from dehydration in combination with other indications such as low urine output

_____ This measure reflects visceral protein status and can indicate nutritional risk when values are less than 3.2 to 3.5

8. TRUE or FALSE (circle one): Upon completion of 3- or 7-day diaries, patients need to record what they ate. The amount of food can be indicated using terms such as "three glasses" of milk, "a scoop of" mashed potatoes, or "a piece" of chicken.

9. The U.S. Department of Agriculture's (USDA) dietary guidelines (https://health.gov/dietary guidelines/2015–2020) include the following (select all responses that are accurate):

_____ 6 oz servings of grains, emphasizing whole grains and higher fiber choices

_____ 2.5 cups of vegetables, emphasis on variety and color

_____ 2 cups of alcoholic beverages with special emphasis on beer and wine

_____ 2 cups from the fat-free or low-fat milk group that also includes fortified soymilk, cheese, yogurt, and tofu

_____ 5 cups of chocolate

_____ 5.5 oz equivalents from the meat and bean group (includes poultry, meats, eggs, and nuts)

_____ 2 cups of fatty fried foods such as french fries or tempura

_____ 5 teaspoons from vegetable oils

_____ 270 calories from discretionary calories including sweets, solid fats, and higher calorie foods

10. TRUE or FALSE (circle one): An examination of the functional integrity of the oral cavity structures is vital for determining the method and type of nutrition a patient can manage.

11. TRUE or FALSE (circle one): The patient's height (length) and weight are the only information needed to determine her/his caloric energy requirements.

12. TRUE or FALSE (circle one): A patient with heart disease was previously placed on a low-fat diet and suffered a stroke one year later associated with onset of significant dysphagia. The patient lost 20 lb within 2 months after stabilizing after the stroke and maintaining the low-fat diet. When addressing the significant weight loss in this patient, it is important to maintain the low-fat diet recommended for managing the heart disease.

13. Daily energy requirements for adults are determined by all of the following EXCEPT
    a. reference to an ideal weight for height in kilograms.
    b. consideration of activity levels or metabolic stressors (e.g., fever, sepsis) that expend more energy.
    c. considering the starting weight of the individual compared with their ideal reference weight.
    d. recommending protein intake of 2.8 g/kg/day.

14. All of the following are <u>TRUE</u> about fluid needs EXCEPT that
    a. generally, adults require 1 mL/kcal of fluid.
    b. fluid needs increase as we age, in general.
    c. fluid needs are typically considered to be proportional to body surface area.
    d. children require 100 mL/kg per day for the first 10 kg of body weight.

15. <u>TRUE</u> or <u>FALSE</u> (circle one): Individuals who aspirate on thin liquid are easily able to maintain adequate hydration levels once prescribed thickened liquids.

16. Noncommercial thickeners that can be used to thicken liquids include
    a. dehydrated potato flakes.
    b. unflavored gelatin.
    c. SimplyThick.
    d. vegetable oil.
    e. Both (a) and (b) are examples of noncommercial thickeners.

17. Match the following nonoral feeding alternatives with their correct definition.
    A. Total parenteral nutrition
    B. Nasogastric tube
    C. Percutaneous endoscopic gastrostomy
    D. Orogastric

    _____ An individual who requires a relatively short duration of tube feeding can have a tube placed through the nose into the stomach through which feeds are administered into the stomach to bypass the upper airway.

    _____ A feeding tube that is placed into the stomach through the mouth using one of two types of tubes, depending on whether the purpose is short term or long term.

    _____ A long-term tube feeding option with the surgical placement of a tube into the stomach so that feeds can be administered directly into the stomach and the tube can be concealed when not in use.

    _____ A patient who cannot take food through the digestive tract is provided her/his nutrition entirely through a large-flow-capacity vein.

14

Pediatric Clinical Feeding Assessment Questions

1. Common etiologies associated with feeding problems in infants and children include the following (select all that apply):

   _____ Sensory deprivation

   _____ Central Nervous System (CNS) disorders (e.g., cerebral palsy, brain malformations)

   _____ Hearing impairment

   _____ Prematurity

   _____ Genetic structural conditions (e.g., cleft palate, Pierre Robin)

   _____ Social-behavioral maladaptation

   _____ Cardiorespiratory compromise

   _____ Gastrointestinal diseases (e.g., esophageal stenosis, gastroesophageal reflux disease [GERD])

   _____ Asthma

   _____ Vaccinations

2. Similar to adult-based dysphagia, pediatric feeding problems can result in the following (select all that apply):

   _____ Malnutrition

   _____ Developmental speech/language delays

   _____ Abnormal suck–swallow–breathe feeding bursts

   _____ Dehydration

   _____ Failure to thrive

   _____ Maintenance of the sucking pads

   _____ Respiratory complications

   _____ Reduced quality of life for caregivers

3. All of the following are signs that an infant or child is aspirating EXCEPT

   a. change in skin color.

   b. wet respiratory sounds.

   c. obstructive inspiratory efforts.

   d. one suck burst per second during nutritive sucking.

4. Long-term consequences of aspiration in pediatric populations include all of the following EXCEPT

   a. stenosis.

   b. bronchiectasis.

   c. tracheal and bronchial granuloma.

   d. recurrent chest infections.

   e. All of the response options are potential consequences.

5. Identify five indications for completing a pediatric clinical feeding assessment.

   a. _____

   b. _____

   c. _____

   d. _____

   e. _____

6. TRUE or FALSE (circle one): Only one observation of the child in a typical clinical exam room will be necessary to obtain representative information regarding typical feeding patterns and problems during a meal.

7. Current popular clinical feeding and mealtime assessment tools available for use include parent questionnaires and observational checklists such as the following (identify four identified within the textbook):

   a. _____

   b. _____

   c. _____

   d. _____

8. Identify the members of a multidisciplinary team for assessing pediatric feeding and swallowing.

_____

_____

9. Medical history information for a pediatric feeding and swallowing evaluation should evaluate _____ and _____ history to obtain details regarding fetal _____, the child's response after delivery, _____, any significant _____ anomalies, and any major _____ during the first few months of life.

10. Prolonged NICU hospitalizations associated with repeated/prolonged tracheal intubations, changes of feeding tubes, and oropharyngeal/tracheal suction episodes may lead to

   a. sensory processing disorders/hypersensitivity.

   b. laryngomalacia.

   c. congenital diseases.

   d. improved feeding outcomes.

11. TRUE or FALSE (circle one): The American Speech-Language-Hearing Association (ASHA) developed a comprehensive, consensus-based set of templates for obtaining a pediatric feeding history and clinical evaluation.

12. TRUE or FALSE (circle one): The family and caregivers involved in the mealtime experience of the child being evaluated do not have valuable information to offer regarding mealtimes, feeding, or medical history of the family and siblings.

13. A current clinical nutritional status can be determined from all of the following EXCEPT

   a. growth chart.

   b. blood count.

   c. anthropometrics.

   d. chemistry panel.

   e. All of the responses above could be used to determine the nutritional status.

14. A child is diagnosed as failing to thrive when

    a. _____

    b. _____

    <u>OR</u>

    c. _____

15. <u>TRUE</u> or <u>FALSE</u> (circle one): There is only one standard growth chart for boys and girls available for reference and use through the CDC at http://www.cdc.gov/growthcharts

16. <u>TRUE</u> or <u>FALSE</u> (circle one): Failure to thrive can be caused by either organic physical causes or nonorganic psychosocial factors, or a combination of these.

17. <u>TRUE</u> or <u>FALSE</u> (circle one): Some children under the 5th percentile are normal—it is the growth trajectory that is often more important as well as consideration of the presence of chromosomal disorders.

18. Feeding history is usually elicited from the _____, _____, _____, or _____.

19. Feeding history should include past methods and patterns of feeding from _____ onward, including _____ to new _____ or textures.

20. The following are important to gather regarding the feeding history EXCEPT
    a. when the feeding problem began.
    b. medical/social circumstances at the time of onset of the feeding problem.
    c. caregiver food preferences.
    d. course of progression of the feeding problem.

21. The caregiver's perception of the following is important to learn during feeding history intake (select all that are correct):

_____ The neonatal history of the parent

_____ Types of foods eaten

_____ Amount of foods eaten

_____ The child's temperature during meals

_____ Textures of foods eaten

_____ Physical environment of meals

_____ Family members present at meals

22. Child readiness for oral feeding can be obtained by all of the following assessment tools EXCEPT the

a. Neonatal Oral–Motor Assessment Scale (NOMAS).

b. Early Feeding Skills Assessment.

c. Feeding Readiness Scale.

d. Eating Assessment Tool (EAT-10).

23. Identify four signs of malnutrition:

a. _____

b. _____

c. _____

d. _____

24. Match each of the following descriptors to the correct contribution to a clinical feeding assessment of the child.

A. Clinical observation

B. Oral sensory–motor assessment

C. Feeding skills assessment

D. Psychosocial–interactional feeding assessment

_____ The child exhibits a prolonged meal duration beyond 30 min.

_____ The child exhibits a rooting reflex upon gentle stroking of the cheek.

_____ The 8-month-old child exhibits aversion to rice cereal during a meal.

_____ The child exhibits a submucosal cleft upon inspection of the hard palate architecture.

_____ The child appears irritable and apathetic.

_____ The parent attempts to place additional food in the child's mouth while the child is still manipulating the last bolus in her/his oral cavity.

_____ The child exhibits oral hypersensitivity.

_____ The child exhibits successful finger feeding and cup drinking.

_____ The child continued to exhibit nutritional suck–swallow patterns at the time the parent thought the child was finished feeding.

_____ The child appears hungry and eager to eat.

_____ The child exhibits age-appropriate gross motor skills.

_____ The child's skin appears abnormally pale.

_____ The child shows a vertical jaw movement during chewing of food.

_____ The child appears anxious in the presence of food.

25. Identify and describe the oral reflexes present in infants that are not present in adults and the typical duration beyond which these disappear during normal development.

a. _____

b. _____

c. _____

d. _____

26. The oral sensorimotor and feeding skills assessment determines _____.

27. Oral reflexes and feeding skills assessments are divided into three infant developmental stages during the first year of life. Assign the following descriptors most appropriate to these three stages:

A. Birth to 4 to 5 months

B. 5 to 7 months

C. 8 to 12 months

_____ Strong rooting reflex during gentle stroking of the cheek

_____ The primary central incisors may be present and lateral incisors erupting

_____ Tongue protrusion reflex in response to food other than liquid on the anterior tongue

_____ Tongue lateralization to manipulate food in the oral cavity is beginning

_____ Drinking from a cup independently

_____ Poor ability to sit upright independently

_____ Starting to open the mouth at the sight of food

_____ Develop a pincer grip on food (hold pieces between the thumb and index finger) during feeding

_____ Stereotypical chewing (vertical jaw motion) and food manipulation are starting

_____ Chewing patterns expand to lateral and possibly rotary movements

_____ Increasingly able to sit independently and hold a bottle or cup

_____ Bite reflex occurs in response to pressure on the anterior or lateral gums

_____ Palmar grasp when picking up food

_____ Insertion of the finger into the mouth triggers a sucking reflex

_____ Primitive reflexes disappear

_____ Anterior–posterior tongue mobility

_____ Beginning to eat solid foods and biting off pieces to chew

_____ Introduction of cereals begins

_____ Oral hypersensitivity in response to foods other than liquids

28. The duration of an infant feeding or child's meal should take no longer than

a. 50 to 60 min.

b. 10 to 15 min.

c. 70 to 75 min.

d. 20 to 30 min.

29. Parent/caregiver and infant/child interactions during a feeding assessment can be evaluated using the _____ developed by the Nursing Child Assessment Satellite Training (NCAST).

a. Parent–Child Feeding Scale

b. Children's Progress Academic Assessment

c. Stanford Binet Intelligence for Young Children

d. Bayley Scales of Infant and Toddler Development

30. TRUE or FALSE (circle one): Premature infants do not have a mature cough reflex such that silent aspiration may be common.

31. Videofluoroscopic assessment of pediatric feeding problems

a. enables observation of the pharyngeal and esophageal phases of feeding.

b. must infer whether aspiration occurred due to limited views of the airway.

c. enables continuous observation of the entire duration of a feeding session.

d. is only used to determine whether the child aspirates or not.

32. All of the following are signs of silent aspiration in a premature infant during feeding EXCEPT

    a. apnea with brachycardia.

    b. obstructive respiratory efforts.

    c. choking/coughing.

    d. cyanosis.

33. <u>TRUE</u> or <u>FALSE</u> (circle one): The use of telehealth for remote pediatric clinical assessment has been validated using a standard remote synchronous-only methodology.

15

Esophageal Phase Dysphagia Questions

1. Match the following structures to their correct location as identified in Figure 15–1.

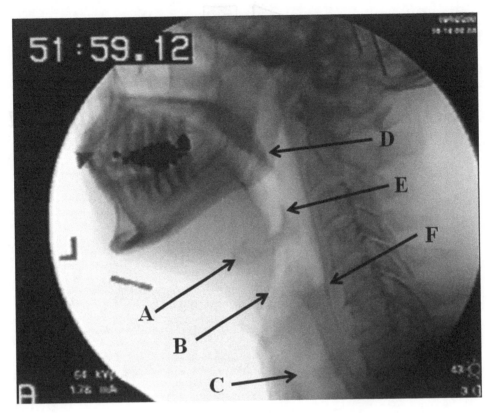

Figure 15-1

_____ Trachea　　　　　　　　_____ Larynx

_____ Soft palate　　　　　　　_____ Hyoid bone

_____ Upper esophageal sphincter　　_____ Epiglottis

2. Match the following structures to their correct location as identified in Figure 15–2.

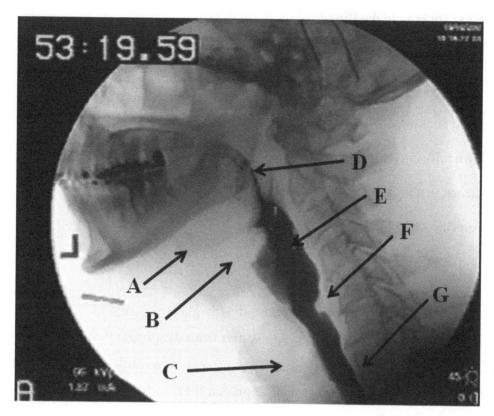

Figure 15-2

_____ Bolus   _____ Upper esophageal sphincter

_____ Esophagus   _____ Oropharyngeal constriction

_____ Larynx   _____ Hyoid bone

_____ Trachea

3. The two regions of the esophagus defined by high pressure generated at rest by the sphincteric muscle are the

a. _____ ; and

b. _____ .

4. Signs and symptoms of dysphagia associated with esophageal etiology include the following (select all that apply):

_____ Food sticking in the throat

_____ Difficulty swallowing liquids

_____ Difficulty swallowing solid foods

_____ Food sticking at the level of the suprasternal notch

_____ Difficulty chewing food

_____ Heartburn or indigestion associated with eating

_____ Sensation of a lump in the throat

_____ Hypernasality

5. The most common cause of esophageal phase dysphagia is _____.

Up to _____% of people with this disease suffer from dysphagia that is likely secondary to

_____ and diminished _____ as a result of chronic inflammation.

The most common and effective treatment approach for this disease is the use of

_____ medication.

6. <u>TRUE</u> or <u>FALSE</u> (circle one): The majority of individuals diagnosed with a hiatal hernia also have dysphagia.

7. Esophageal inflammation associated with dysphagia can be caused by the following (select all that apply):

_____ *Candida albicans*

_____ Tracheostomy

_____ Chemoradiation therapy

_____ Food allergies

_____ Colon cancer

_____ Foreign body/pill impaction

8. The definitive procedure for diagnosing infectious esophagitis is

   _____

9. All of the following are risk factors for esophageal candidiasis EXCEPT
   a. diabetes mellitus.
   b. immunodeficiency.
   c. oropharyngeal dysphagia.
   d. history of chemotherapy/radiation therapy.
   e. corticosteroid use.

10. Medications may systemically cause esophageal dysphagia by

    a. _____
    b. _____
    c. _____

11. Medication may DIRECTLY cause esophageal dysphagia by

    _____

    _____

12. Methods that can be used to reduce or prevent direct esophageal mucosal injury include

    a. _____
    b. _____
    c. _____
    d. _____

13. Individuals diagnosed with eosinophilic esophagitis may have a prior history of

    a. _____
    b. _____
    c. _____

14. Eosinophilic esophagitis may be characterized by the following (select all that apply):

    _____ "Trachealized," or ringed, appearance to the esophagus during endoscopy

    _____ Solid food dysphagia

    _____ Dysarthria

    _____ Esophageal strictures

    _____ Esophageal food impactions

    _____ Vocal fold paralysis

    _____ <20 eosinophils per high-powered field view on biopsy

    _____ Normal-appearing esophageal mucosa

15. One difference between a Schatzki A-ring and B-ring is the location of each relative to the _____ junction. An A-ring is a thick muscular ring typically found at the upper border of the _____ sphincter, whereas the B-ring is a membranous ring typically found at the _____ junction.

16. The preferred treatment of a Schatzki A-ring is _____ injection into the muscular ring. Esophageal _____ is typically unsuccessful. A Schatzki B-ring exhibits a contrast in esophageal mucosa on either side with _____ mucosa on the proximal margin and _____ mucosa on the distal margin. This type of ring is successfully treated with _____.

17. Unlike Schatzki rings, esophageal _____ are characterized by mucosal constrictions in the esophagus above the gastroesophageal junction. These exhibit _____ mucosa on both the proximal and distal margins and occur in the _____ portion of the esophagus. The optimal treatment for these constrictions is esophageal _____.

18. Abnormal pressure generation and its patterns can also cause problems characterized as ineffective esophageal _____. The best means for diagnosing these forms of esophageal dysphagia require the use of _____.

19. The following are examples of esophageal dysphagia etiologies characterized by impaired patterns of esophageal pressure generation for bolus propulsion (select all that apply):

_____ Schatzki rings

_____ Hypertensive lower esophageal sphincter (LES)

_____ Distal esophageal spasm (DES)

_____ Eosinophilic esophagitis

_____ Achalasia

_____ Nutcracker esophagus

_____ Gastroesophageal reflux disease (GERD)

20. The most common esophageal motor abnormality in individuals diagnosed with GERD is _____. This disorder is characterized by low-amplitude (<30 mm Hg) peristaltic esophageal contractions in more than 30% of manometrically tested swallows.

21. Define the following esophageal motility disorders.

a. Esophagogastric junction outflow obstruction:

_____

_____

_____

_____

b. Nutcracker esophagus:

_____

_____

_____

_____

c. Distal esophageal spasm:

_____

_____

_____

_____

d. Achalasia:

_____

_____

_____

_____

22. All of the following are considered to be autoimmune etiologies of esophageal dysphagia EXCEPT

a. scleroderma.

b. Parkinson disease.

c. Sjögren syndrome.

d. All of the above are correct.

23. Select all of the following statements that are true of neoplasms associated with esophageal dysphagia.

_____ Esophageal tumors are rarely malignant.

_____ Squamous cell carcinoma is a frequent tumor type associated with esophageal cancer.

_____ The least common esophageal tumor type is adenocarcinoma.

_____ Papillomas and cysts are examples of benign esophageal tumors.

_____ Patients often can localize the site of esophageal neoplasms.

_____ Esophagoscopy is recommended for complaints of solid food dysphagia to rule out esophageal neoplasms.

24. Esophageal motility disorders are defined as an abnormality of _____

    outflow and/or derangement of _____. It is important to rule out a/an

    _____ abnormality using esophagoscopy. In the absence of apparent mucosal

    or structural abnormalities, _____ is frequently the next step to

    understand and visualize esophageal physiologic function. If inconclusive, supportive

    diagnostic testing includes conventional timed _____ with concurrent

    13-mm barium tablet and/or the functional lumen imaging probe (FLIP) system.

25. The functional lumen imaging probe (FLIP) system is used to

    a. evaluate oropharyngeal physiology.

    b. measure maximum pharyngoesophageal segment opening during swallowing.

    c. quantify the directionality of upper esophageal sphincter opening.

    d. quantify the degree of opening and compliance of the lower esophageal sphincter (LES).

    e. All of the above are correct responses.

26. All of the following may be used to classify the cause of a primary esophageal motility
    disorder EXCEPT

    a. esophagogastric junction outflow obstruction (EGJOO).

    b. proximal esophagus spasm (PES).

    c. distal esophagus spasm (DES).

    d. ineffective esophageal motility (IEM).

    e. All of the above are correct responses.

16

Neurogenic Dysphagia Questions

1. More than 75% of those with oropharyngeal dysphagia are represented by _____ disorders.

2. The ability to accurately identify aspiration in an individual with neuromyogenic conditions during a bedside evaluation (clinical evaluation of swallowing) ranges from _____ to _____% sensitivity and _____ to _____% specificity due to their risk of _____ aspiration. Sensitivity represents the proportion of individuals identified <u>WITH</u> or <u>WITHOUT</u> (circle one) dysphagia who are <u>CORRECTLY</u> or <u>INCORRECTLY</u> (circle one) identified as such, and specificity represents the proportion of individuals identified <u>WITH</u> or <u>WITHOUT</u> (circle one) dysphagia who are <u>CORRECTLY</u> or <u>INCORRECTLY</u> (circle one) identified as such.

3. The two best instrumental methods for identifying the presence or absence of silent aspiration in those with neuromyogenic etiologies of dysphagia are

   a. _____

   b. _____

4. Individuals suffering a stroke are at risk for dysphagia. During acute stages after stroke onset, up to _____% exhibit dysphagia. At 1 year poststroke, between _____ and _____ % exhibit chronic dysphagia associated with malnourishment and _____, the most common cause of rehospitalization in acute stroke patients and the cause of death in _____% of individuals within the first 30 days poststroke.

5. Following a stroke, the optimal timing for speech-language pathology assessment of dysphagia is within three

   a. days.

   b. weeks.

   c. months.

   d. years.

6. Match the following signs and symptoms of dysphagia following stroke with their respective affected CNS counterpart.

A. Nucleus ambiguus

B. Hypoglossal nucleus

C. Cortical activation of the facial nucleus

D. Cortical activation of the hypoglossal nucleus

E. Superior laryngeal nerve, or nucleus tractus solitarius

_____ Pharyngeal weakness

_____ Facial asymmetry and weakness

_____ Silent aspiration

_____ Tongue asymmetry and fasciculations

_____ Tongue deviation away from the side of cortical damage with normal symmetry and tone of the tongue

_____ Difficulty forming a cohesive bolus

_____ Weak cough

7. Select all of the following conditions typically found associated with dysphagia in individuals diagnosed with Parkinson disease.

_____ Difficulty initiating a swallow

_____ Increased difficulty swallowing liquids compared to solid foods

_____ Prolonged pharyngeal transit

_____ Hyperkinesia

_____ Tongue pumping (several posterior tongue movements prior to triggering a swallow)

_____ Normal esophageal motility

_____ Delayed airway protection relative to bolus transit

8. Amyotrophic lateral sclerosis (ALS) is a neurodegenerative disease with presentation of both _____ and _____ motor neuron impairment. It is common to observe tongue _____ and _____ as well as onset of _____ pneumonia.

9. Select all of the following that are characteristic of a patient with traumatic brain injury.

    _____ Evidence of primitive reflexes (tongue pumping, sucking, tongue extrusion)

    _____ Only occurs in adults

    _____ Impaired coordination of oropharyngeal movements

    _____ Respiratory function requiring a tracheostomy or ventilator

    _____ Normal cognitive function

    _____ Delayed onset of swallowing

    _____ Injury to cortical and subcortical structures

    _____ Impaired lower motor neurons

10. Multiple sclerosis is characterized by upper and lower motor neuron impairment due to the formation of _____ on nerve sheaths resulting in impaired neural _____. With progression of this disease dysphagia <u>IMPROVES</u> or <u>WORSENS</u> (circle one).

11. The Dysphagia in Multiple Sclerosis (DYMUS) questionnaire is divided into two scales that provide good internal validity and reliability for screening individuals with multiple sclerosis. The two scales on this instrument screen for dysphagia with _____ and _____ foods.

12. Cerebral palsy (CP) is a neurological motor and processing disorder arising in childhood. A hallmark characteristic of this disorder is muscle _____.

13. Depending on the severity and range of associated impairments, muscle spasticity in people with CP may affect deglutition for all of the following reasons (select all that apply).

_____ Abnormal posture   _____ Laryngeal penetration/aspiration

_____ Impaired oral stage function   _____ Hemifacial paralysis

_____ Tongue fasciculation   _____ Impaired mastication

14. Individuals with dementia and Alzheimer's disease exhibit impaired memory and cognitive decline. The most common cause of death in this population is _____. Poor cognition, poor memory, and inability to _____ all contribute to eating impairment.

15. Many elderly individuals take multiple _____ that can cause _____ and exacerbate dysphagia. Some individuals have difficulty swallowing _____ requiring reformulation of medications to liquids for improved swallowing safety. To test this ability, it is recommended during a DSS protocol to evaluate the ability of elderly individuals to swallow a _____ mm _____.

16. Polymyositis, dermatomyositis, and inclusion body myositis are examples of _____ that occur when _____.

17. Due to prolonged pharyngoesophageal narrowing, or obstruction, the proximal pharynx may respond by increasing muscle activation or might result in pharyngeal dilatation as evident by the presence of a hypopharyngeal _____.

18. The most common form of muscular dystrophy in newborn males is _____, caused by a genetic defect that prevents production of the muscle protein _____.

19. Oculopharyngeal muscular dystrophy is most commonly associated with _____ dysfunction in 75% of affected individuals. Early identification and treatment of the latter may prevent eventual formation of pharyngeal _____, or hypopharyngeal _____.

20. Myotonic dystrophy (MD) is associated with dysphagia most frequently affecting the _____ and _____ with aspiration detected in over _____% (Willaert et al., 2015).

21. Myasthenia gravis is an autoimmune disorder characterized by _____ _____ _____. The hallmark symptom of myasthenia gravis during an activity is _____. Thus, rehabilitative exercises are not recommended to treat dysphagia. Rather, treatment of dysphagia usually utilizes _____ and _____.

22. Identify all of the following muscular dystrophies with their correct description.

    A. Oculopharyngeal

    B. Myotonic

    C. Duchenne

    _____ The most common of the muscular dystrophies, which does not occur until adulthood. It is associated with progressive muscle wasting and weakness with impact on swallowing affecting the pharynx and upper esophageal sphincter most.

    _____ This disease is caused by a genetic defect for the protein in muscles called dystrophin, resulting in rapid worsening of the disease. It affects boys rather than girls due to the pattern of inheritance such that girls are carriers only. Onset is usually prior to the age of 6 years.

    _____ This disease is inherited and typically does not occur until middle age with onset of eyelid drooping (ptosis) initially followed by onset of swallowing difficulties related to pharyngeal weakening.

17

Dysphagia in Head and Neck Cancer Patients Questions

1. TRUE or FALSE (circle one): Chemotherapy is unlikely to be associated with dysphagia because it does not cause changes in the affected tissues other than to reduce or eliminate the tumor.

2. TRUE or FALSE (circle one): Patients with laryngeal or hypopharyngeal tumors are more likely to aspirate prior to treatment than those with tumors in the oral cavity or oropharynx.

3. The best predictor of long-term swallowing function in head and neck cancer patients is PRE-/POST- (circle one) treatment swallowing function.

4. A study by Langerman et al. (2007) determined that aspiration was observed prior to treatment in _____% of those with oral cavity tumors, in _____% of those diagnosed with cancer in the oropharynx, and in _____% of those with cancer in the hypopharynx.

5. Identify two tumor characteristics that have been found to be predictive of dysphagia severity prior to treatment of head and neck cancer.

   a. _____

   b. _____

6. TRUE or FALSE (circle one): It is optimal to complete a swallowing assessment after initiation of head and neck cancer treatment due to the unlikely occurrence of pretreatment dysphagia and the accuracy by which clinicians can rely on patient self-report.

7. Identify the four methods used to treat cancer affecting structures of the head and neck.

   a. _____

   b. _____

   c. _____

   d. _____

8. The musculature of the floor of the mouth is primarily responsible for

   a. _____

   b. _____

9. Consequences of surgical treatment of the floor of the mouth for head and neck cancer may include the following:

    a. _____

    b. _____

    c. _____

    d. _____

    e. _____

    f. _____

    g. _____

10. Select all of the following dysphagia side effects that may occur associated with chemotherapy.

    _____ Odynophagia

    _____ Nasal regurgitation

    _____ Mucositis

    _____ Impaired tongue mobility

    _____ Anorexia

    _____ Impaired pharyngeal constriction

    _____ Xerostomia

    _____ Infections in the oral and pharyngeal cavities

    _____ Oronasal fistula and nasal residual

11. Surgical treatment for cancer affecting the lips can impair the following eating functions:

    a. _____

    b. _____

    c. _____

    d. _____

12. Select all of the following dysphagia side effects that may occur associated with surgical treatment.

_____ Odynophagia

_____ Nasal regurgitation

_____ Pseudoepiglottis

_____ Improved cough efficacy

_____ Reduced or absent hyolaryngeal excursion

_____ Posterior pharyngeal wall tethering during swallowing

_____ Impaired tongue mobility

_____ Loss of smell

_____ Blindness

_____ Oronasal fistula and nasal residue

_____ Impaired pharyngeal constriction

_____ Improved airway closure

_____ Xerostomia

_____ Increased jaw range of motion

13. Select all of the following dysphagia side effects that may occur associated with radiation treatment.

_____ Mucositis

_____ Odynophagia

_____ Drooling

_____ Reduced or absent general sensation

_____ Reduced or absent hyolaryngeal excursion

_____ Impaired tongue mobility

_____ Pharyngeal residue

_____ Impaired pharyngeal constriction

_____ Enhanced mandibular mobility

_____ Silent aspiration

_____ Fibrosis of soft tissues

_____ Weight gain

_____ Pharyngoesophageal stenosis

14. During chemoradiation, placement of a feeding tube may be recommended either prophylactically or during a course of treatment to

a. _____

b. _____

c. _____

15. Match the following descriptions with the correct surgical procedure.

   A. Total laryngectomy

   B. Supraglottic laryngectomy

   C. Partial laryngectomy

   D. Base of skull

   E. Mandibulectomy

   _____ Removal of the mandible

   _____ Only the laryngeal structures invested with cancer are removed and reconstruction of the remaining tissues involved in voice production, typically requiring a permanent tracheostomy due to inadequate airway opening

   _____ Removal of cancer involving the superior portion of the larynx such as the ventricular and aryepiglottic folds, epiglottis, and hyoid bone

   _____ Removal of a tumor near the jugular foramen involving the CNs IX and X or in the infratemporal fossa

   _____ Removal of the entire larynx and reconstruction of its attachments within the pharynx, including creation of a permanent tracheostomy to separate the airway from the esophagus

16. TRUE or FALSE (circle one): Evaluation of deglutition after surgical treatment for head and neck cancer should be planned beyond 7 to 10 days or more after surgery to allow the patient time to heal at the site of the surgical deficit before assessing the impact on her/his eating function.

17. Dysphagia related to the acute effects of radiation therapy may continue for

   _____ (duration) beyond completion of treatment. Due to the effect of

   radiation on soft tissues, patients may experience _____,

   resulting in decreased or absence of hyolaryngeal elevation and tongue mobility.

18. The rationale for using chemoradiation treatment as the first approach for a head and neck cancer rather than surgery and radiation is

_____

_____

_____

Long term, dysphagia in patients treated using this approach is FREQUENT or INFREQUENT (circle one) as the intensity of these treatments has INCREASED or DECREASED (circle one) to improve treatment outcomes.

19. The three most common dysphagia findings reported in head and neck cancer patients treated with chemoradiation include the following:

    a. _____

    b. _____

    c. _____

20. Intensity modulated radiation therapy was developed to INCREASE or DECREASE (circle one) radiation scatter so that it concentrates the radiation on the _____. Unfortunately, pharyngeal dysphagia may still result because the _____ constrictors continue to receive a high degree of radiation, resulting in impaired function. Even in patients with survival beyond 1 year reported to be eating a normal oral diet, 26% exhibited _____ and 60% of those with the latter exhibited _____ and ineffective _____ (Feng et al., 2010). Thus, patient perception of function after chemoradiation treatment may be CONSISTENT or INCONSISTENT (circle one) with findings from more objective evaluation of deglutition.

21. Match the following treatment approaches used in those with head and neck cancer with their targeted dysphagia pathophysiology.

    A. Masako exercise: Instruct patients to stick out their tongue and hold it between their lips or teeth while they swallow.

    B. Effortful swallow: Instruct patients to swallow as hard as they can during a saliva or bolus swallow using an analogy like, "swallow like you would when you need to swallow a large vitamin without water."

    C. Shaker exercise: Instruct patients to lie in a supine position and to lift and hold their head upward while looking toward their toes for 60 s while maintaining contact between their shoulders and the floor, or mat. Patients can then lower their head and repeat this 30 times with an eventual goal of three sets of 30 head lifts.

    _____ This method is used to recruit as many motor units as possible during swallowing in those with weakened oropharyngeal musculature, particularly those with difficulty swallowing their secretions or with excess saliva production.

    _____ This method is used to enhance recruitment of pharyngeal constrictor muscle activation during swallowing by reducing participation of the base of tongue in oropharyngeal constriction during swallowing.

    _____ This method is used to improve reduced superior and anterior excursion of the hyolaryngeal complex associated with piriform sinus residue.

22. The goals of clinicians managing individuals with head and neck cancer are

    a. PHYSICIAN GOAL:

    _____

    _____

    b. SPEECH-LANGUAGE PATHOLOGIST GOAL:

    _____

    _____

23. Individuals with head and neck cancer frequently have difficulty with eating associated with their cancer treatment. When this occurs, a feeding tube is placed for the purpose of

    a. _____

    b. _____

18

Laryngopharyngeal Reflux Questions

1. The definition of laryngopharyngeal reflux (LPR) is

   _____

   _____

2. Laryngopharyngeal reflux (LPR) can cause the following (select all that are correct):

   _____ Dysphonia

   _____ Gastroesophageal reflux disease (GERD)

   _____ Laryngeal granulomas

   _____ Nasopharyngeal cancer

   _____ Subglottic stenosis

   _____ Asthma

3. As few as _____ (#) LPR reflux episodes per week appear adequate for damaging laryngeal tissue with a preexisting mucosal condition according to a study completed by Koufman in 1991.

4. Assign the letter to each of the following characteristics that best describes (A) GERD versus (B) LPR.

   _____ Heartburn

   _____ Esophagitis

   _____ Daytime reflux

   _____ Nighttime reflux

   _____ Reflux occurs in supine position

   _____ Reflux occurs in upright position

   _____ Prolonged episodes of reflux

   _____ Brief episodes of reflux

   _____ Body mass index increases prevalence

   _____ Body mass index does not increase prevalence

   _____ Lower esophageal sphincter dysfunction is an etiology

   _____ Esophageal dysmotility is not an etiology

   _____ Upper esophageal sphincter dysfunction is an etiology

5. <u>TRUE</u> or <u>FALSE</u> (circle one): Laryngeal tissues are well equipped to withstand exposure to gastric refluxate components such as acid and pepsin, unlike esophageal tissues.

6. Of the nine items on the Reflux Symptom Index (Belafsky et al., 2002), these were found to be the most common complaints of individuals diagnosed with LPR (select all that apply):

   _____ Hoarseness or a problem with your voice

   _____ Clearing your throat

   _____ Excess throat mucus or postnasal drip

   _____ Difficulty swallowing food, liquid, or pills

   _____ Coughing after you ate or after lying down

   _____ Breathing difficulties or choking episodes

   _____ Troublesome or annoying cough

   _____ Sensations of something sticking in your throat or a lump in your throat

   _____ Heartburn, chest pain, indigestion, or stomach acid coming up

7. Endoscopic findings associated with LPR include the following (select all that apply):

   _____ Vocal fold edema   _____ Papilloma

   _____ Granuloma/granulation   _____ Thick endolaryngeal mucus

   _____ Vocal fold paresis/paralysis   _____ Pseudosulcus (infraglottic edema)

   _____ Ventricular obliteration   _____ Vocal fold hemorrhage

   _____ Erythema/hyperemia   _____ Posterior commissure hypertrophy

   _____ Diffuse laryngeal edema

8. Define the following terms.

   a. Pseudosulcus:

   _____

   _____

   _____

   _____

   b. Reinke's space edema:

   _____

   _____

   _____

   _____

   c. Vocal fold granuloma:

   _____

   _____

   _____

   _____

9. The gold standard for diagnosing LPR is _____. Placement of the upper probe should be <u>ABOVE</u> or <u>BELOW</u> (circle one) the upper esophageal sphincter so that it <u>IS</u> or <u>IS NOT</u> (circle one) in the proximal esophagus. The lower probe should be placed 5 cm <u>ABOVE</u> or <u>BELOW</u> (circle one) the lower esophageal sphincter. Esophageal _____ is recommended to assure desirable probe placement. Endoscopic visualization <u>DOES</u> or <u>DOES NOT</u> (circle one) ensure confirmation of lower probe placement. Diagnosis of LPR is made by considering the presence or absence of _____ injury and the number of reflux events in the hypopharynx at a pH of _____ or less given the pH level necessary to activate pepsin.

10. The presence or absence of LPR may also be more common in the presence of a devastating form of esophageal cancer known as _____.

11. Lifestyle modifications frequently recommended to treat reflux include the following (select all that apply):

    _____ Avoid alcoholic beverages

    _____ Avoid lying down less than 3 hr after eating

    _____ Prop your head up during sleeping by 4 in.

    _____ Eat fatty foods

    _____ Avoid acidic foods such as citrus and tomatoes

    _____ Eat larger meals frequently

    _____ Stop smoking

    _____ Bring weight to normal standards

    _____ Eat chocolate and peppermint

    _____ Elevate the head of the bed by 6 in,

    _____ Avoid wearing tight clothing

12. <u>TRUE</u> or <u>FALSE</u> (circle one): Chewing gum can increase pH levels in the esophagus and pharynx by stimulating salivary bicarbonate production and repeated swallowing, making this a desirable behavior.

13. The position of the American Academy of Otolaryngology–Head and Neck Surgery is that LPR treatment requires the prescription of _____

    <u>ONCE</u> or <u>TWICE</u> (circle one) daily to suppress gastric acid for longer than _____ hr. In addition, they recommend this regimen for more than _____ months for LPR symptom improvement and more than _____ months for improvement of laryngeal findings. These medications should also be taken _____ to _____ min prior to meals for maximum efficacy.

14. In severe and life-threatening cases of LPR, surgical treatment may be recommended. LPR symptoms have been shown to improve after _____ or _____.

19

Spinal Abnormalities in Dysphagia Questions

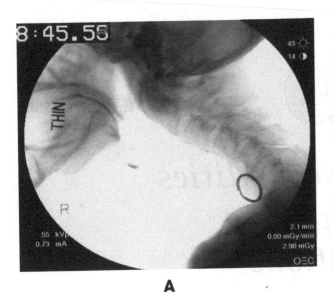

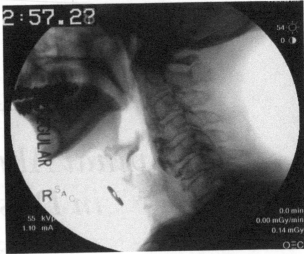

A   **B**

1. Refer to figures A and B:

   Figure A shows an example of an individual with a cervical spine having excessive <u>CONVEX</u> or <u>CONCAVE</u> (circle one) curvature of the cervical spine consistent with <u>KYPHOSIS</u> or <u>LORDOSIS</u> (circle one). Figure B shows an example of an individual with <u>LORDOSIS</u> or <u>OSTEOPHYTES</u> (circle one) affecting the lower cervical vertebral column.

2. The occurrence of osteophytes was identified in the Japanese population (Teraguchi et al., 2014) in _____% of those younger than age 50 and in _____% of those older than age 50. The most commonly affected cervical vertebrae across all studied were _____.

3. Select all of the following that could explain the underlying pathophysiology of dysphagia in someone with cervical osteophytes.

   _____ Narrowing of the pharyngeal diameter

   _____ Impaired soft palate elevation

   _____ Bolus obstruction in the upper esophageal sphincter (UES) or esophagus

   _____ Poor oral bolus transit

   _____ Impeded epiglottic inversion

4. <u>TRUE</u> or <u>FALSE</u> (circle one): The key factor in onset of dysphagia subsequent to cervical spinal surgery is the occurrence of injury to the vagus nerve.

5. Postoperative dysphagia following cervical fusion is typically associated with
   a. plate thickness.
   b. multilevel plating.
   c. fusion to C3–C4.
   d. None of the above responses.
   e. All of the above responses.

6. Traction diverticuli are considered to be a late postoperative development after cervical neck fusion. These:
   a. occur as lateral pouches in the pharynx.
   b. progressively form within the pharyngeal mucosa and submucosa.
   c. are the result of a delayed ischemic nerve injury.
   d. are the same thing as a Zenker's diverticulum.

7. Symptoms of dysphagia remaining chronic were associated with worsening of _____ and _____ in a study by Leonard and Belafsky (2011).
   a. pharyngeal constriction ratio, pharyngoesophageal segment opening
   b. pharyngeal transit time, epiglottic inversion
   c. pharyngeal transit time, hyoid elevation
   d. pharyngeal wall thickness, aspiration

8. Smith-Hammond et al. (2004) showed that _____% of individuals undergoing anterior spinal surgery developed dysphagia, whereas _____% of those undergoing posterior cervical spinal surgery developed dysphagia. _____ percent of those undergoing lumbar spinal surgery developed dysphagia.

9. Identify all of the following comorbidities that need to be ruled out before attributing dysphagia solely to cervical spine abnormalities.

_____ Neurodegenerative disease

_____ Cerebrovascular accident

_____ Cricopharyngeus muscle dysfunction

_____ Incontinence

_____ Pregnancy

_____ GERD

10. TRUE or FALSE (circle one): Cervical spinal surgery patients exhibit reduced reflux symptomatology indicative of improved control of stomach acid.

11. Match each of the following dysphagia management approaches with the targeted pathophysiology.

A. Sensory stimulation

B. Masako exercise

C. Progressive lingual resistance exercises

D. Reduced bolus size

E. Increased bolus size

F. Lubrication of foods

_____ Reduced UES opening during the swallow

_____ Reduced base of tongue motion

_____ Reduced pharyngeal muscle function

_____ Solid food dysphagia with narrowed pharynx due to obstructive pathology

_____ Poor epiglottis deflection

_____ Delayed swallow onset, or reduced sensation to bolus residue

12. When spinal abnormality is severe enough to significantly impact deglutition, surgical options include _____ to remove osteophytes or _____ in situations where cervical hardware significantly limits epiglottic inversion. However, when comorbidities or patient status precludes surgical intervention, _____ feeding may be the preferred option.

Bonus Online-Only Chapter 🖱ⓦ

Telehealth

The workbook includes a Bonus Online-Only Chapter based on the accompanying textbook chapter on telehealth for the management of dysphagia. This bonus chapter will include similar activities designed to facilitate learning and the application of telehealth-related knowledge and skills important to clinicians implementing this modality of service delivery as well as students in clinical training programs. This Bonus Online-Only Chapter can be accessed on the PluralPlus companion website.

Answers

CHAPTER 1: ANATOMY AND PHYSIOLOGY OF DEGLUTITION ANSWERS

1. a. **Deglutition:** The entire act of eating that includes putting a food substance or liquid in the mouth, its preparation for swallowing, oropharyngeal swallow, and transport of the bolus through the esophagus ending with the bolus entering the stomach.

   b. **Feeding:** Placement of food or liquid in the mouth, manipulation of food or liquid in the oral cavity prior to the swallow, and the oral stage of deglutition, including the oral transit of food from the oral cavity into the pharynx.

   c. **Mastication:** Characterized by chewing and manipulation of a bolus within the oral cavity that requires contributions from the tongue, jaw, and lips. This is a volitional act.

   d. **Swallowing:** This is characterized by a series of sequential structural movements that propels food or liquid through the pharynx and esophagus into the stomach. Swallowing occurs through a nearly stereotypical sequence of movements of structures resulting in constriction behind the bolus and dilation ahead of the bolus associated with a positive pressure behind the bolus and a drop in pressure ahead of the bolus, respectively. Once triggered, the swallow cannot be stopped volitionally, rendering it to be a nonvolitional response.

   e. **Bolus:** A formed mass of liquid or food that is ingested.

   f. **Aspiration:** Material passes through the vocal folds into the lower airway.

   g. **Laryngeal penetration:** A term that refers to the entry of a bolus into the laryngeal vestibule.

   h. **Residue:** Material remaining in the oral cavity, pharynx, or esophagus after a swallow.

   i. **Dysphagia:** Impaired ability to feed or eat that can include impaired ability to suck, chew, swallow, or clear food from the oral cavity, throat, or esophagus during eating. Additional problems can include difficulty placing food in the mouth, controlling saliva, taking oral medications, or coughing/choking related to meals. Pediatric populations may show difficulty breastfeeding, bottle feeding, drinking from a cup, eating from a fork or spoon, or chewing.

2. __B__ Propulsion of the bolus into the pharynx

   __A__ Mastication of the bolus

   __D__ Transportation of the bolus through the esophagus to the stomach

   __A__ The bolus is mixed with saliva

   __C__ Transportation of the bolus through the pharynx into the esophagus

   __C__ Airway closure occurs associated with cessation of respiration

   __B__ The soft palate begins to elevate as the posterior tongue depresses

   __D__ Bolus propulsion occurs through coordinated peristaltic contraction of both smooth and striated muscle

3. d. frontal.

4. a. Vomer

   b. Ethmoid (perpendicular plate)

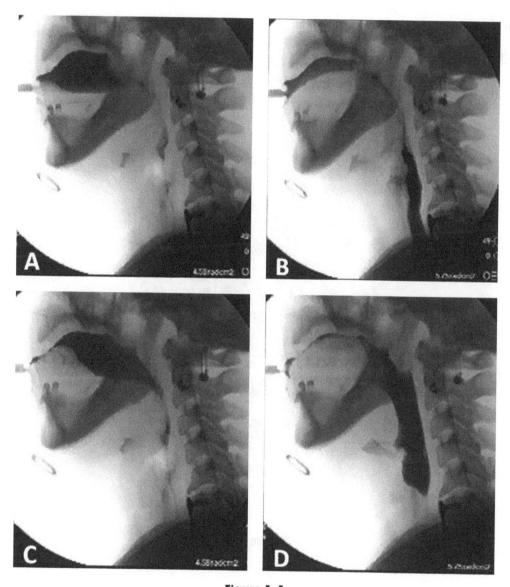

Figure 1-1

5. __A__ Preparatory   __D__ Pharyngeal

   __C__ Oral   __B__ Esophageal

6. c. Palatine

   d. Maxilla

7. c. Ethmoid

8. Frontal, parietal, occipital, temporal, sphenoid, ethmoid

9. Mandible; temporomandibular joint

10. C5–C6

11. Mandible, maxilla, palatine

12. Ethmoid; cribriform plate

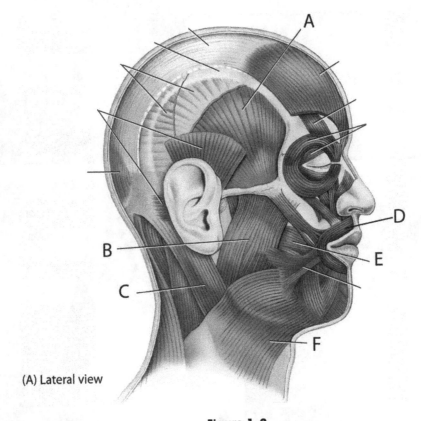

(A) Lateral view

Figure 1-2

13. A Temporalis

    B Masseter

    C Sternocleidomastoid

    D Orbicularis oris

    E Buccinator

    F Platysma

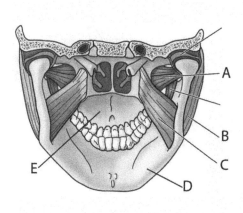

(D) Posterior view of viscerocranium

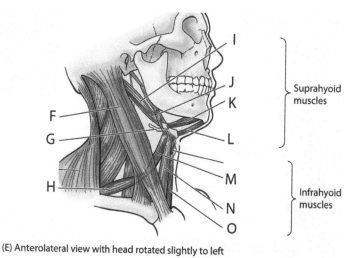

Suprahyoid muscles

Infrahyoid muscles

(E) Anterolateral view with head rotated slightly to left

Figure 1-3

14. A Lateral pterygoid muscle

B Masseter muscle

C Medial pterygoid muscle

D Mandible bone

E Maxilla bone

F Sternocleidomastoid muscle

G Hyoid bone

H Inferior belly of the omohyoid muscle

I Posterior belly of the digastric muscle

J Stylohyoid muscle

K Anterior belly of the digastric muscle

L Geniohyoid muscle

M Superior belly of the omohyoid muscle

N Sternohyoid muscle

O Sternothyroid muscle

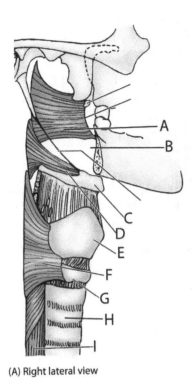

(A) Right lateral view

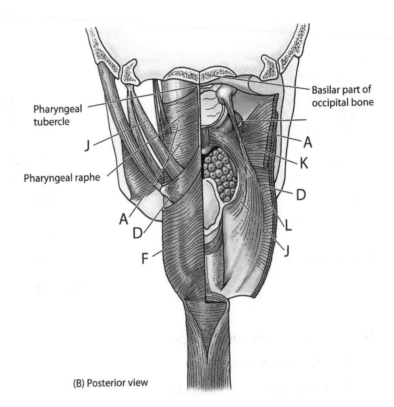

Pharyngeal tubercle

Pharyngeal raphe

Basilar part of occipital bone

(B) Posterior view

Figure 1–4

15. A   Superior constrictor muscle

    B   Mandible bone

    C   Hyoid bone

    D   Middle constrictor muscle

    E   Thyroid cartilage

    F   Inferior constrictor muscle

    G   Cricoid cartilage

    H   Trachea

    I   Esophagus

    J   Stylopharyngeus muscle

    K   Salpingopharyngeus muscle

    L   Palatopharyngeus muscle

16. Masseter muscle (internal and external; CN V); temporalis (CN V); and medial (internal) pterygoid (CN V)

17. Lateral (external); pterygoid (CN V)

18. a. Palatoglossus

    b. Palatopharyngeus

19. __X__ Normal salivary secretion ranges from 1.0 to 1.5 L per day.

    __X__ Saliva contains an enzyme for digesting starches.

    __X__ Saliva controls pathogenic bacteria responsible for dental caries.

    __X__ Saliva contains mucus for lubrication.

20. Levator palatini (pharyngeal plexus of CN X [vagus])

21. Orbicularis oris and buccinator muscles; innervation for both is from CN VII (facial)

22. Superior, middle, and inferior constrictor muscles

23. The <u>thyropharyngeus</u> contributes to the hypopharynx, or laryngopharynx. This muscle remains at resting length and constricts during the pharyngeal swallow. The <u>cricopharyngeus</u> contributes to the upper esophageal sphincter and remains constricted until a pharyngeal swallow is triggered. At that time, the cricopharyngeus relaxes so that the upper esophageal sphincter can be stretched during hyolaryngeal excursion so that it opens to allow a bolus to pass into the esophagus.

24. Superior longitudinal, inferior longitudinal, transversus, verticalis; innervation is from the hypoglossal nerve (CN XII)

25. Palatopharyngeus

26. Thyroarytenoid, cricothyroid, lateral cricoarytenoid, and interarytenoid

27. Posterior cricoarytenoid

28. True vocal folds, ventricular folds (i.e., false folds), and aryepiglottic folds

29. Mylohyoid

30. Mylohyoid, anterior digastric, medial and lateral pterygoids, geniohyoid, stylohyoid, styloglossus, posterior tongue, superior constrictor, palatoglossus, and palatopharyngeus

31.
G	Levator veli palatini	G	Palatopharyngeus
A	Tensor veli palatini	A	Anterior digastric
B	Orbicularis oris	B	Posterior digastric
B	Buccinator	A	Masseter
I	Styloglossus	A	Temporalis
H	Superior constrictor	A	Medial pterygoid
H	Middle constrictor	A	Lateral pterygoid
H	Inferior constrictor	F	Thyroarytenoid
A	Mylohyoid	J	Sternohyoid
B	Stylohyoid	E	Cricothyroid
I	Geniohyoid	I	Thyrohyoid
G	Palatoglossus	F	Posterior cricoarytenoid

32.
C	Taste to the anterior two-thirds of the tongue
D	Taste to the posterior one-third of the tongue
B	General sensation to the oral cavity
D	General sensation to the faucial pillars
B	General sensation to the face and lips
E	General sensation to the oro- and laryngopharynx (a.k.a., hypopharynx)
E	General sensation to the laryngeal vestibule and surface of the vocal folds
G	General sensation to the inferior portion of the vocal folds and trachea
A	Sense of smell

33. Lateral regions of the primary motor cortex and the premotor areas

34. Internal capsule, subthalamus, amygdala, hypothalamus, substantia nigra, mesencephalic reticular formation, monoaminergic brainstem nuclei, and the corticofugal swallowing pathway

35. __X__ Consists of a group of neurons within the reticular formation of the brainstem

__X__ Receives afferent input from the trigeminal (V), glossopharyngeal (IX), and vagus (X) nerves

__X__ Triggers a swallow pattern in response to stimulation of the superior laryngeal nerve branch of the vagus nerve (SLN)

__X__ Includes the nucleus tractus solitarius as the principal sensory nucleus involved in triggering the coordinated motor output

__X__ Includes coordination of a complex sequence of motor output from the hypoglossal (XII) nucleus and nucleus ambiguus (X) to produce the oropharyngeal swallow

__X__ Interneurons within the ventral swallowing group serve to distribute and coordinate activation of the motor neurons activated during swallowing

__X__ Trigeminal and hypoglossal motor nuclei are only connected to interneurons within the ventral swallowing group

__X__ Bilateral coordination of motoneuron pools is thought to occur via interneurons within the trigeminal and hypoglossal motor nuclei

36. esophagus.

37. Relaxation of the cricopharyngeus and hyolaryngeal excursion (the hyoid bone and larynx move vertically and anteriorly due to contraction of suprahyoid and extrinsic laryngeal muscles, resulting in opening of the pharyngoesophageal segment where the upper esophageal sphincter resides).

38. Upper esophageal sphincter (i.e., pharyngoesophageal segment) and lower esophageal sphincter

39. TRUE

FALSE

TRUE

TRUE

FALSE

FALSE

FALSE

TRUE

TRUE

FALSE

40. The internal superior laryngeal nerve branch of the vagus nerve (CN X, SLN branch) is not responsive to the presence of food within the laryngeal vestibule, placing Susan at risk for aspiration. Other signs could suggest that Susan has aspirated silently without triggering the recurrent laryngeal nerve branch of the vagus nerve (CN X, RLN branch), such as an elevated temperature after eating (i.e., spiking a fever), frequent occurrence of upper respiratory infections, or a history of aspiration pneumonia.

41. Stan has a serious respiratory disorder and struggles to maintain oxygen levels during tidal breathing that worsens during physical exertion, including eating; therefore, it is likely that Stan's coordination of breathing and swallowing is impaired, placing him at risk for aspiration pneumonia.

CHAPTER 2: HEAD AND NECK PHYSICAL EXAM ANSWERS

1. __X__ I cough and choke during meals.

   __X__ I feel like there is something in my throat after I eat and I have to clear my throat to get it out.

   __X__ My voice changes when I eat and I sound gurgly.

   __X__ My child refuses to eat and cries during meals.

   __X__ Food sticks in my throat.

   __X__ It hurts when I swallow.

   __X__ It takes me about an hour to finish a meal because I need to take small bites and chew my food really well.

   __X__ I only eat soup or drink protein drinks because meat and vegetables stick in my throat.

2. a. anatomic structures.

   b. motor function.

   c. sensory function.

3. a. determining the patient's chief complaint and symptoms.

   b. discussing the patient's past and relevant medical history.

   c. a head and neck examination.

4. __D__ Heartburn, indigestion, or feeling a lump in the throat

   __A__ Dry mouth (xerostomia)

   __E__ Reduced range of motion of the jaw after radiation therapy (trismus)

   __F__ Coughing and choking during meals

   __B__ Breathy voice quality, lose air quickly when talking

   __C__ Food sticks in my throat that needs to be cleared by drinking water

5. REDUCE

   XEROSTOMIA

6. INCREASE

   DROOLING

7. REDUCE

   XEROSTOMIA

8. REDUCE

   XEROSTOMIA

9. TRUE

10. Impact communication due to sticking of articulatory structures; promote mucosal damage; predisposition to dental caries; increased risk of serious respiratory infection due to loss of antimicrobial activity of saliva; impaired ability to masticate food; difficulty initiating the swallow and clearing food from the oral and pharyngeal cavities; impaired sense of taste; oral discomfort, particularly for denture wearers; denture misfit; and consequent predisposition to malnutrition

11. __X__ Symmetry of the face

　　 __X__ Sensitivity of the tongue to touch

　　 __X__ Movement of the lips and eyelids

　　 __X__ Signs of drooling

　　 __X__ Sense of taste and smell

　　 __X__ Range of jaw motion during mouth opening

　　 __X__ Eye movements and pupil function

　　 __X__ Sensitivity of the face to touch

12. __X__ Tongue symmetry and tone

　　 __X__ Elevation of the soft palate during phonation

　　 __X__ Tongue protrusion and other movements

　　 __X__ Sense of taste

　　 __X__ Voice quality during phonation

　　 __X__ Hyolaryngeal elevation during a swallow

　　 __X__ Gag response

13. TRUE

14. a. indirect laryngoscopy using a head light and a mirror.

　　 b. endoscopic examination using a flexible nasoendoscope (sometimes, they may also use a rigid scope to perform stroboscopic examination of the vocal folds).

15. __X__ Examination of the nasal passageways

　　 __X__ Velopharyngeal integrity and function during speech and swallowing

　　 __X__ Base of tongue integrity and behavior during breathing, swallowing, and speech

　　 __X__ Masses or tumors within the naso-, oro-, and laryngopharyngeal regions

　　 __X__ Sensation of the oro- and hypopharyngeal structures

　　 __X__ Oropharyngeal and hypopharyngeal clearance of boluses after a swallow

　　 __X__ Oropharyngeal and hypopharyngeal bolus residue after a swallow

CHAPTER 3: CLINICAL SWALLOW EVALUATION ANSWERS

1. A swallow screening is an abbreviated test to determine whether an individual is at risk for having dysphagia, is aspirating, or can eat safely by mouth. If an individual does not pass the swallow screening, they require a comprehensive clinical swallow evaluation that includes a thorough review of their medical and feeding history, physical examination of the oral–motor and respiratory anatomy and function, and observation of swallowing to determine whether additional imaging or other instrumental studies are needed and to formulate a treatment strategy.

2. **Water swallow tests:** Administration of a known quantity of water with the instruction to drink it as quickly as possible and to observe whether coughing occurs or a change in voice quality during or after completion of the swallow. If coughing or a voice change occur during testing, additional monitoring or referral for instrumental examination will be recommended.

   Toronto Bedside Swallowing Test (TOR-BSST): This screen combines an oral exam, motor tasks, and an initial assessment as to whether the individual is alert, can speak clearly, and swallow versus observed signs of weakness.

   Cervical auscultation: Involves recording or listening to swallowing sounds using a stethoscope or laryngeal microphone. The examiner listens for variations from what is considered a normal pattern in the series of typical sounds associated with a swallow to determine abnormal swallowing patterns or aspiration. This method has been reported to have mixed results in successfully identifying abnormal sounds of swallowing, but has been more useful in identifying abnormal respiratory sounds associated with aspiration.

   Pulse oximetry: This method uses a monitor typically placed on the index finger to detect changes in arterial blood oxygenation in response to aspiration. This method is sometimes combined with the water swallow test, but it has been studied with mixed results.

3. __X__ Pulmonary history suggestive of aspiration

   __X__ Unexplained weight loss

   __X__ Malnutrition or dehydration

   __X__ Caregiver or patient concerns are expressed regarding swallowing problems

   __X__ Dysarthria and a gurgly voice quality

4. FALSE

5. a. Adequate oral control of the bolus

   b. Adequate clearance of the bolus from the oral cavity, pharynx, and esophagus

   c. Respiratory coordination with the swallow to ensure airway safety

   d. Adequate airway protection before and during the swallow

   e. Normal executive functions

6. FALSE

7. TRUE

8.
B	Weight gain	A	Drooling
A	Chronic obstructive pulmonary disorder	B	Head tilting to assist in getting food to the throat to swallow
A	Carotid artery surgery	B	Dysarthria
B	Non-English speaker	A	Uncuffed trach tube in place
A	Base-of-tongue cancer	B	Hearing loss
B	Developmental speech abnormality	A	Fed by caregiver
A	Tube feedings	A	Cerebral palsy
B	Normal oral diet	A	Stroke
B	Complete a meal within 30 min	A	Hiatal hernia
A	Choking on liquids	A	Food residue in the oral sulci
A	Regurgitation of food 1 hr after eating	A	Poor dentition and oral hygiene
B	Likes to talk during meals	A	Excessively dry mouth
A	Sensation of a lump in the throat	B	Prefers to eat meat and potatoes
B	Appropriately responds to questions and follows instructions	B	Has a twin
A	Food sticks in the throat at the level of the larynx	A	Completed radiation therapy to the head or neck
B	Radiating pain down the left arm during running	B	Poor vision
A	Gradual increase in sticking of food in the throat after 65 years of age	A	Difficulty swallowing pills

9. Gloves, small flashlight, tongue blades, small laryngeal mirror, feeding apparatus (cups, spoons, syringe and catheter, pipette), food and liquid (e.g., ice chips, water, thick liquid, puree, cracker, or other similar solid such as a shortbread cookie, saltine cracker, or graham cracker), emesis basin, washcloth, towel or paper towels, cotton swabs, gauze, gauze rolls, flexible straws, coffee beans, peppermint, lemon juice, sugar water and saline for testing taste, and suction.

10.
X	Medical and surgical history
X	Past and current medications
X	Swallowing history
X	Respiratory status assessment
X	Physical examination of the oral mechanism

___X___ Evaluate articulatory precision and rate

___X___ Sensation to taste of sugar, salt, or lemon

___X___ Assessment of patient cognitive status and alertness

___X___ Assess signs of aspiration during swallowing of food and liquid

___X___ Oropharyngeal reflex testing

11. a. Hypotheses should relate to signs of cranial nerve impairment related to Mr. Jones's left cortical stroke manifesting in impaired function of muscles innervated by CN VII and CN XII as follows:

TONGUE MOBILITY IMPAIRMENT: Mr. Jones exhibits signs of impaired tongue mobility as indicated by his imprecise articulation of anterior lingual sounds and deviation of his tongue to the right during protrusion. Given the symmetry of the tongue and appearance of intact tone in the context of a left CVA, it is possible that Mr. Jones exhibits an upper motor neuron lesion of the hypoglossal nerve (CN XII). Difficulty manipulating the ice chip such that it was lost to the pharynx and possibly aspirated indicates impairment to the oral prep phase of deglutition associated with right-sided impairment of the tongue, although further evaluation of the lingual-palatal valve should be tested to rule out oral preparatory volitional control problems versus impaired integrity of the lingual–palatal valve (see 11.b. section).

LOWER QUADRANT OF THE RIGHT FACIAL MUSCLES IMPAIRED: Mr. Jones shows asymmetry and drooling from the right side of the mouth suggestive of lower right quadrant weakness of facial musculature. This would also be consistent with an upper motor neuron lesion to the facial cranial nerve (CN VII) associated with Mr. Jones's left CVA.   Impaired lip seal as a result of lower right facial weakness may affect deglutition by impairing the ability to keep food in the mouth and possibly contributing to a site of pressure loss during onset of oral transit and oropharyngeal swallowing.

b. It remains unclear whether Mr. Jones's loss of the ice chip was related to poor anterior lingual control, reduced sensation to the tongue, or poor posterior oral cavity seal between the base of the tongue and soft palate. Given the likelihood of an upper motor neuron lesion to CN XII and VII, it is unlikely that taste and general sensation are impacted as those would require a lower motor neuron impairment. However, the case description did not state whether sensory function was tested. It is important to address this in order to build the case regarding an upper motor neuron impairment versus a lower motor neuron impairment. Similarly, it is important to test sensorimotor function of the pharynx to determine the patient's risk of aspiration. To test these hypotheses, the following can be done:

   i. Test general sensation (CN V) to the upper-face, mid-face, and lower-face regions externally and also to the oral cavity. Use a cotton swab to touch the left and right portions of the skin overlying the forehead, cheeks, mandible, lips, anterior 2/3 of the tongue dorsum, buccal mucosal lining of the cheeks, and also the hard palate while Mr. Jones closes his eyes.

   ii. Test general sensation to the anterior faucial pillar (CN IX).

iii. Test general sensation associated with triggering the gag response (CN X, pharyngeal plexus) by touching a tongue blade to the posterior tongue, posterior faucial pillar, and posterior pharyngeal wall.

iv. Test sensation to taste by administering saline solution, sugar solution, and lemon juice via a cotton Q-tip swab to the left and right portions of the anterior portion of the tongue (CN VII), and ask Mr. Jones to identify what he tastes while he sticks out his tongue. (If he retracts his tongue, it might contaminate the posterior tongue, which is innervated for taste by CN IX.)

v. Assessment of the facial symmetry and tone was reported already (rest observation). However, information regarding assessment of lip strength in holding a seal upon command was not reported. Thus, the patient should puff out his cheeks with air to determine if he can sustain air in his oral cavity with a lip seal. Next, application of pressure to the cheeks would determine how strong this seal is. Nonspeech movement assessment of the lips to determine symmetry and range of movements is important to confirm differences in left and right lip function.

vi. Symmetry in jaw position at rest was not reported but is hypothesized to be normal if the etiology of observed problems relates to upper motor neuron impairment to cranial nerves VII and XII. Rest observation of the jaw needs to be assessed as well as strength and range of motion during nonspeech movements such as opening the mouth widely and then closing the jaw. Lateral jaw movements can be assessed as well as the ability of the patient to open his mouth against resistance and to close his mouth against resistance.

vii. The observation of resting tongue symmetry and tone was already reported. In addition to sensory testing, volitional nonspeech movements should be tested. If the tongue impairment is isolated to the genioglossus, deviated tongue protrusion away from the site of lesion (left cortical stroke) is expected to be the primary impairment with reduced tongue strength in lateral or protrusive movements made against resistance using a tongue blade. However, other tongue movements such as elevation (inside and outside of the oral cavity), retraction, and lateral movement toward the site of lesion would be expected to be performed with normal range of motion and strength.

viii. Speech testing of the tongue was not reported and can be completed by conducting diadochokinetic testing of lingual movements during speech production of "puh-puh-puh," "tuh-tuh-tuh," and "kuh-kuh-kuh" syllables during 7 s durations to test which are impaired for precision and rate. Additional testing of syllable combinations can also be completed. Impaired production of "tuh" is expected given the observation that Mr. Jones exhibits impaired articulation of anterior lingual sounds; however, impaired production of the "kuh" syllable could indicate poor elevation of the base of the tongue that may be associated with losing the ice chip to the pharynx before onset of swallowing. It should also be noted whether Mr. Jones exhibits hypernasality on oral plosive speech sounds indicative of velopharyngeal insufficiency, possibly indicative of impaired elevation of the soft palate.

ix. Observation of Mr. Jones's soft palate was also reported during rest observation and during sustained phonation of "ah." The observations indicated normal function of the velopharynx during speech production. However, if the testing proceeds to food testing, it will be important to determine whether liquids travel through the nasal passage, suggesting impaired closure of the velopharynx during swallowing. Given that velopharyngeal function is controlled bilaterally by the cortical hemispheres, a lower motor neuron impairment is expected to result in impaired function of this structure.

x. Laryngeal function can be tested by asking Mr. Jones to first try to hold his breath for 10 s. In some instances, individuals may feel they are holding their breath by simply not exhaling. Thus, it is important to ensure that Mr. Jones is holding his breath at the larynx level by asking him to push air out slightly while holding his breath. Also note his breathing rate to ensure it is at a normal pace or if his respiratory status places him at risk for abnormal breathing patterns surrounding a swallow. Next, ask him to sustain phonation of "ah" for as long as possible to complete auditory–perceptual assessment of his voice quality and vocal efficiency. If his voice sounds breathy or raspy, it may indicate that his vocal folds are not functioning normally. If his voice sounds gurgly, it may suggest that saliva is accumulating in his laryngeal vestibule. In the latter situation, it is important to note whether Mr. Jones exhibits sensitivity to the presence of secretions in his laryngeal vestibule by throat clearing or coughing to clear materials. If there is no response to a gurgly voice quality, this may imply impaired function of the internal branch of the superior laryngeal nerve (internal SLN, CN X). If he demonstrates throat clearing or coughing in response to materials in his laryngeal vestibule, this would be considered a sign of intact supraglottal sensation for elicitation of a protective response. Mr. Jones was reported to cough in response to administration of an ice chip that was lost from his oral cavity, suggesting that he has intact sensitivity to the ice chip entering the airway. Given that direct observation through imaging was not available at the time, it remains unclear whether the ice chip merely penetrated into the laryngeal vestibule or was aspirated. If aspirated, it may be the case that he did not respond until the ice chip entered the trachea, which indicates intact function of the recurrent laryngeal nerve. Next, it is important to note the integrity and strength of Mr. Jones's cough. If he exhibits a strong productive cough, then it is likely he effectively cleared the airway of the ice chip. That said, without imaging, it remains unknown how effective Mr. Jones is in clearing materials that penetrate the larynx or are aspirated from the description of his case. Based on the hypotheses proposed, it is anticipated that Mr. Jones exhibits a strong productive cough and minimal voice impairment, if any.

xi. It is also possible that Mr. Jones has been nil per os (NPO) for a week and his first try with the ice chip did not go well because he has not been eating anything by mouth. Prior to administering additional ice chips, it is a good idea to administer oral hygiene to clean Mr. Jones's oral cavity to minimize the risk of aspiration of oral bacteria that may put him at risk for aspiration pneumonia. Thereafter, administration of a series of ice chips and observing whether Mr. Jones exhibits improved control of the ice chip for swallowing assessment can be done.

xii. If Mr. Jones exhibits improved progression with the ice chips, testing with small quantities of water can then be completed, and so forth, until it is determined what the limit of oral swallowing for Mr. Jones currently is.

c. The clinical evaluation will allow determination of Mr. Jones's risk for problems with deglutition involving the oral cavity versus the pharyngeal phase. If Mr. Jones exhibits problems that appear isolated to the oral cavity and no signs of aspiration are determined, it may be possible to work with Mr. Jones to minimize oral-related problems by manipulating bolus placement in the oral cavity or exploring other approaches for managing oral preparatory and oral phase bolus management challenges. In these cases, Mr. Jones should be instructed to hold his breath to protect the airway in advance of administration of an ice chip or water bolus. If successful, it may be recommended that Mr. Jones can begin to have ice chips and water after completion of oral hygiene. However, if the patient exhibits signs of pharyngeal impairment or aspiration, then additional testing using videofluoroscopy or endoscopy is warranted to determine the underlying problem so that a treatment plan can be proposed. The decision to remain NPO should be made with consultation of Mr. Jones's physician and be based on his respiratory and health status. If he shows risk of aspiration, it may be recommended to introduce oral hygiene prior to administration of ice chips and water. However, if his respiratory and health status is compromised, he may need to remain NPO until additional testing can be completed.

CHAPTER 4: ENDOSCOPY IN ASSESSING AND TREATING DYSPHAGIA ANSWERS

1. __X__ The patient needs a same-day bedside evaluation.

   __X__ A swallowing evaluation in the clinic is needed.

   __X__ Need to rule out impaired mobility and range of motion of pharyngeal anatomy.

   __X__ There are concerns regarding radiation exposure for the patient.

   __X__ Need to test the foods typically eaten by the patient.

   __X__ Need to observe secretions within the pharynx and their buildup over several swallows.

   __X__ Laryngeal and pharyngeal sensitivity are questioned and need evaluation.

   __X__ Need to observe the coordination of bolus flow and airway protection.

   __X__ Would like to use biofeedback during swallowing maneuvers.

   __X__ Need to directly evaluate the impact of swallowing maneuvers and positions.

2. e. Only (a) and (c) are possible.

3. c. is observed to penetrate the laryngeal aditus into the laryngeal vestibule but does not penetrate below the vocal folds.

4. d. lips.

5. b. Sustained phonation of /s/

6. FALSE

7. c. touch the epiglottis or arytenoid mucosa with the scope tip.

8. f. All of the above.

9. a. the ice chip protocol.

10. b. ask the patient to hold a liquid bolus in the oral cavity to the count of three before initiating the swallow.

11. d. All of the above.

12. __6__ Test positional, compensational, and swallowing maneuver techniques and observation of impact

    __4__ Administration of mechanically soft boluses

    __2__ Administration of a small liquid bolus

    __1__ Examination of the pharyngeal anatomy and movements

___5___ Administration of solid foods, including mixed consistencies

___3___ Administration of increasingly larger liquid boluses

13. FALSE

14. FALSE

15. b. incorporates sensory testing of the pharynx and larynx.

16. ___X___ Secretions pooling on the vocal folds

___X___ Buildup of secretions in the left piriform sinus

___X___ Immobility of the right vocal fold

___X___ Increased size of the left ventricular fold such that it obstructs most of the left vocal fold view

17. d. All of the above.

CHAPTER 5: BARIUM RADIOGRAPHIC EVALUATION OF THE PHARYNX AND ESOPHAGUS ANSWERS

1. a. **Cineradiography:** This procedure entails recording the motion picture onto individual frames of a motion picture film from the output portion of a fluoroscopic image intensifier into a camera. The frames are then played back at a rate that allows visual perception of a smooth and fluid movement as was originally seen during the recording.

   b. **Videofluoroscopy:** This procedure is similar to cineradiography with the exception that the moving picture is recorded at a rapid rate onto a videotape or digital disk from a monitor receiving the output images from the fluoroscopic image intensifier.

   c. **Ultrasound:** Also referred to as sonography, high-frequency sound waves are sent outward and then transduced into images based on the pressure waves returning. The transducer is placed onto a gel that maximizes conductance of the sound pressure waves through the skin overlying the region of soft tissues of interest. Ultrasound is used to observe the anatomy and movement of soft tissue structures such as internal organs, muscles, and tendons. This method does not use X-rays, and this reduces radiation exposure. The patient can sit upright while eating during this procedure.

   d. **Computed tomography:** Computed tomography (CT) is a specialized type of radiographic imaging approach that acquires a series of cross-sectional images from the region of the body where the structure of interest is located. Each cross-sectional image results from a computational reconstruction of multiple angles of images taken as an X-ray beam rotates around the individual's body at the location of the structure of interest. The thickness of the imaged sections can be as small as 1 mm. Advancements in this method of imaging to achieve high-resolution reconstructed images allow helical or spiral scanning methods in addition to the original axial method. In addition, the use of an electron beam can be used without having to move portions of the scanner. This procedure exposes the patient to radiation; the typical CT is conducted with the patient supine, but upright positioning is achieved in a standing CT.

   e. **Magnetic resonance imaging:** This method does not expose the patient to radiation, as images are obtained by way of a powerful magnet in which the patient lies in a supine position. The magnetic field of the magnet is used to change the alignment of atomic nuclei in the body to cause a rotating magnetic field from tissues in the body that can be reconstructed into an image. Soft tissues can be contrasted from each other using this method.

2. 1

   INADEQUATE

3. cumulative

   IS NOT

4. c. hertz.

5. __X__ Peak voltage across the X-ray tube (kVp)

   __X__ Tube current × exposure time (milliampere seconds, mAs)

   __X__ Image field size

   __X__ Source distance to the skin surface

   __X__ Source distance to the detector

   __X__ Use of a grid

   __X__ Screening time in advance of recording

6. d. All of the above are true.

7. TRUE

8. c. It is the same as an esophagram.

9. a. determine symmetries or asymmetries in bolus pathway and clearance.

10. FALSE

11. c. total pharyngeal transit time.

12. esophageal phase

   20-

   stomach

   tablet

   stomach

   70

13. aortic arch

   mainstem bronchus

14. a. **Reflux:** This refers to the movement of stomach contents backward into the esophagus and sometimes up to the laryngopharynx.

   b. **Trendelenburg position:** This position is often used during radiographic evaluation of esophageal function. In this position, the individual is laid in the supine position with the feet raised or higher than his/her head from 15° to 30°.

   c. **Valsalva maneuver:** This maneuver refers to the effort to exhale while closing off the airway. This can be done by closing the mouth and pinching the nose or by closing the larynx while bearing down.

d. **Secondary peristalsis:** This term refers to observation of peristaltic esophageal contractions that occur after the primary peristaltic wave and occur in response to retention of material in the esophagus requiring additional clearance.

e. **Tertiary esophageal contractions:** This term refers to contractions occurring in the distal third of the esophagus that do not cause propulsion of a bolus.

CHAPTER 6: DYNAMIC FLUOROSCOPIC SWALLOW STUDY: SWALLOW EVALUATION WITH VIDEOFLUOROSCOPY ANSWERS

1. c. monitor an individual while he/she eats a meal.

2. FALSE

3. __X__ Radiation exposure limits testing duration to less than 5 min

   __X__ Utilizes a standard protocol rather than observation of a typical meal

   __X__ Cannot test sensation of tissues

   __X__ Implementation of radiopaque contrast boluses

   __X__ Individual must sit upright and be mobile

4. a. Patient respiratory history and physical status relevant to tolerance for the procedure and fragility

   b. The patient's performance on oral, pharyngeal, and laryngeal tasks during the clinical evaluation of swallowing

   c. The effects of diseases and/or their prior interventions on deglutition

   d. The cognitive and behavioral condition of the patient that might affect his/her ability to respond appropriately to commands or participate in the activities of the DSS

5. __X__ So that each patient's performance on the DSS can be compared with those of others

   __X__ To compare performance on the DSS over time or from pre- to posttreatment

   __X__ To ensure consistency in DSS performance across clinicians

   __X__ To compare performance on different types of tests of deglutition (e.g., FEES, manometry)

6. The anterior portion should include the lips, and the posterior view should include the palate and a portion of the nasopharynx as well as the atlas portion of the cervical spine. The inferior–posterior view should contain the cervical esophagus. This view will also provide images that contain the trachea, pharynx, larynx, hyoid bone, tongue, mandible, and floor of mouth.

7. a. measurement of pharyngeal transit time.

8. FALSE

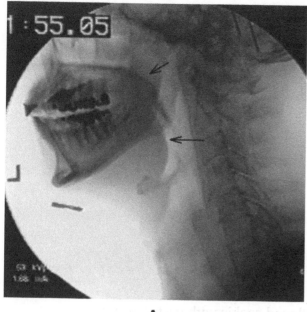

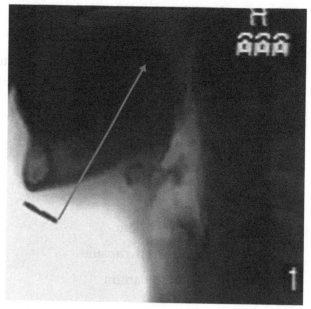

A   **B**

9. A

    B

    FALSE

10. __C__   Position of the patient/upper airway structures

    __G__   Postural stability/flexibility

    __B__   Respiratory sufficiency

    __I__   Stamina and endurance

    __A__   Lubrication

    __D__   Bolus characteristics

    __F__   Competing behaviors and states

    __E__   Environment

    __H__   Adaptability

    __J__   Imaging views

11. __X__   Enables comparison of findings from pre- to posttreatment

    __X__   Enables comparison of findings to normative data

    __X__   Improves testing consistency between and within clinicians and institutions

    __X__   Reduces radiation exposure due to the efficiency with which information is gathered

12. TRUE

13. **LATERAL VIEW:**

_____3_____ 20-cc bolus of liquid barium

_____5_____ 1/4 of a shortbread cookie with paste barium

_____2_____ 3-cc bolus of liquid barium

_____6_____ 60-cc liquid barium via straw drinking

_____1_____ 1-cc bolus of liquid barium

_____4_____ 3-cc paste barium

A/P VIEW:

_____1_____ 3-cc paste barium

_____3_____ 13-mm barium capsule

_____2_____ 20-cc liquid barium

14. d. chewing and swallowing a quarter of a shortbread cookie with paste barium.

15. FALSE

16. TRUE

17. d. All of the above.

18. _____X_____ Modified bolus consistency

_____X_____ Modified bolus volume

_____X_____ Modified bolus placement within the oral cavity

_____X_____ Bypassing the oral cavity with a syringe or catheter

_____X_____ Preswallow breath holding

_____X_____ Head/neck flexion

19. _____X_____ Use a nipple with a slower rate of release

_____X_____ Position the infant in a less supine position during feeding

CHAPTER 7: DSS: A SYSTEMATIC APPROACH TO ANALYSIS AND INTERPRETATION ANSWERS

1. c. evaluation of how well the patient progressed through his/her typical meal.

2. b. fluoroscopic frame size.

3. TRUE

4. TRUE

5. c. poor bolus containment in the oral cavity during oral preparation.

6. b. reduced hyolaryngeal excursion.

7. FALSE

8. a. with the head and neck in a neutral position.

9. linguapalatal

   base of the valleculae

10. e. All of the above.

11. respiration

    airway

    linguapalatal

    velopharyngeal

    aryepiglottic fold (laryngeal)

12. d. Both (a) and (b) are correct, but (c) is not.

13. FALSE

14. FALSE

15. TRUE

16. e. Both (b) and (d) are correct.

17. d. the presence of a Schatzki A-ring.

18. bolus residue can build up within the piriform sinuses and eventually spill into the airway when the larynx is open during respiration, resulting in aspiration.

19. IS

20. pharyngeal constriction

    anterior/posterior

21. hyolaryngeal

    upper esophageal sphincter

22. d. Only (a) and (c) are correct.

23. __X__ Aspiration prior to laryngeal closure may be due to delayed triggering of the swallow.

     __X__ Aspiration prior to laryngeal closure may be due to impaired linguapalatal valving.

     __X__ Aspiration during maximum laryngeal closure is due to impaired laryngeal closure.

     __X__ Aspiration after or between swallows is due to residue falling into the airway once the larynx reopens.

24. a. a normal voice quality.

25. d. Both (a) and (c) are correct, but not (b).

26. TRUE

27. TRUE

28. FALSE

29. b. the timing of the PES opening should be considered delayed based on bolus arrival in the hypopharynx.

30. FALSE

31. A/P

    STANDS UPRIGHT

    20-mL

    LIQUID

    MOTILITY

    STRUCTURAL ABNORMALITY

CHAPTER 8: DYNAMIC SWALLOW STUDY: OBJECTIVE MEASURES AND NORMATIVE DATA IN ADULTS ANSWERS

1. FALSE

2. TRUE

3. TRUE

4. f. All of the above.

5. f. The only correct statements are (a) and (c).

6. FALSE

7. c. determine the presence/absence of pneumonia.

8. FALSE

9. TRUE

10. k. Both (a) and (h) are incorrect examples of bolus transit times.

11. d. All of the above.

12. FALSE

13. __G__ The duration of time between approximation of the epiglottis against the arytenoid cartilage (AEclosure) and return of the epiglottis to preswallow position (Em)

__D__ The time at which the PES closes associated with the tail of the bolus fully in the esophagus; this gesture defines the end of the oropharyngeal swallow

__A__ The time at which airway closure occurs during the swallow is associated with onset of the initiation of elevation of the aryepiglottic folds (AEstart) and the time at which the downward folding of the epiglottis (AEclose) makes contact with the arytenoid cartilages

__F__ The duration of time between the first opening of the PES and PES closure

__C__ The time at which the PES appears to open associated with entry of the bolus head

__E__ The time at which the epiglottis appears to return to the preswallow position; this gestural time marks full restoration of an open respiratory status following a discrete swallow

__B__ The initiation of superior-anterior displacement of the hyoid bone (H1) associated with a swallow followed by the time at which the hyoid bone reaches its maximum superior-anterior excursion during the swallow (H2); the time at which the hyoid shows its first return movement to rest position (H3) also allows measurement of the total duration of time taken associated with hyoid displacement during the swallow

14. b. H2.

15. c. The time of the first movement of the hyoid bone in the anterior-superior direction

16. __D__ The duration of time from PES opening to PES closing (Pcl–Pop)

__C__ The total time between the oropharyngeal and hypopharyngeal transit times (BP2–B1)

__A__ The duration of the bolus transit through the oropharynx as measured from the point in time when the bolus passes the posterior nasal spine (B1) to the time the bolus exits from the valleculae (BV2)

__F__ The duration of maximum hyoid displacement as measured from the point of maximum anterior-superior displacement during the swallow until the hyoid bone initiates a return to preswallow position (H3–H2)

__E__ The duration of supraglottic airway closure during the swallow indicated by the time from arytenoid cartilage approximation to the epiglottis until the epiglottis returns to preswallow position (Em–AEc)

__B__ The duration taken for the bolus to transit through the hypopharynx as measured from the time the bolus head initiates exit from the valleculae (BV2) to the time the bolus tail clears the PES (BP2)

17. FALSE

18. __T__ As the size of the bolus increases, the duration of PES opening (Pcl–Pop) increases.

__T__ As bolus size increases, the duration of PES opening increases.

__F__ As bolus size increases, the total duration of oropharyngeal swallow also increases.

__F__ The duration of hyoid bone maximum displacement is longer during swallows of paste than for 3-cc liquid boluses.

__T__ The duration of PES opening is prolonged during swallows of a paste bolus than for liquid boluses.

__F__ The duration of airway closure (Em–AEclose) is longer during smaller bolus sizes than larger bolus sizes.

__T__ The duration of maximum hyoid bone displacement (H3–H2) is reduced in elderly individuals (>65 years) without dysphagia compared with younger normal individuals for 1-cc, 3-cc, and 20-cc liquid bolus sizes.

19. __X__ Initiation of airway closure indicated by elevation of the aryepiglottic folds (AEstart) always begins prior to PES opening (Pop).

__X__ The PES always closes at the same time or just after the bolus tail clears the sphincter (BP2).

__X__ Onset of UES opening (Pop) always occurs before the time of maximum hyoid to larynx approximation (HLx).

20. __B__ This spatial measure defined as the referent position of deglutition structures while the individual holds a 1-cc bolus in the oral cavity

__D__ The width at maximum distention of the PES during the swallow as a liquid bolus passes through

__A__ The maximum anterior to superior change in hyoid bone position from referent hold position

__E__ The distance between the larynx and hyoid bone during their maximum approximation during the swallow

__C__ The ratio of pharyngeal area measured in the lateral view at the point of maximum constriction during the swallow divided by the pharyngeal area in the referent hold position

21. TRUE

22. FALSE

23. __8__ HLm: The timing of maximum approximation of the hyoid bone and larynx

__2__ B1: The onset of supraglottal closure indicated by movement of the arytenoid cartilage elevation and downfolding of the epiglottis

__3__ H1: The head of the bolus having reached the base of the valleculae

__10__ BP2: The timing of the tail of the bolus clearing the PES

__9__ PAm: The timing of maximum pharyngeal constriction

__3__ BV1: The head of the bolus beginning to exit from the valleculae

__5__ BP1: The timing of the hyoid bone at its maximum superior-anterior excursion during the swallow

__10__ Pcl: The timing of the first closure of the PES closing on the tail of the bolus

__4__ AEc: The time at which the PES appears open

__2__ AEs: The first superior-anterior displacement of the hyoid that results in a swallow

__3__ BV2: The epiglottis approximating the arytenoid cartilages, indicating supraglottal closure

__5__ Pop: The head of the bolus first entering the UES as it opens

__6__ H2: The timing of the maximal opening of the PES

__1__ ONSET: The first movement of the bolus past the posterior nasal spine

__7__ PESm: The timing of maximal distension of the UES

24. ___X___ The older individual showed a delayed onset of the swallow compared with the younger individual.

    ___X___ The older individual exhibited pharyngeal residue after the first swallow, whereas the younger individual did not exhibit pharyngeal residue.

    ___X___ The older individual showed reduced pharyngeal constriction compared with the younger individual.

25. FALSE

26. a. can help explain reduced PES opening in some patients with dysphagia as the elevation of the hyoid and larynx contribute to this swallow gesture.

27. c. is considered to reflect information relevant to airway protection and PES opening during the swallow.

28. TRUE

29. b. larger in individuals older than 65 years compared with those younger than 65 years.

30. FALSE

31. ___T___ PESmax has been shown to be reduced in elderly (>65 years) compared with younger (≤65 years) individuals.

    ___F___ The maximum displacement of the hyoid bone (Hmax) has been shown to be reduced in elderly (>65 years) compared with younger (≤65 years) individuals.

    ___F___ Bolus size has been found to affect measures of the distance between the hyoid bone and the larynx during maximum approximation during the swallow, with the larger distance associated with larger bolus sizes.

    ___T___ The maximum opening of the pharyngoesophageal segment (PESmax) has been found to increase with increased bolus size.

    ___T___ Increased bolus sizes have been associated with increased displacement of the hyoid bone at its maximum displacement (Hmax).

32. ___X___ An association was found between impaired PES function and pharyngeal dilation and weakness as indicated by increased measures of pharyngeal area during the referent hold position (PAhold) associated with decreased opening of the PES (PESmax).

    ___X___ Investigation of pharyngeal changes after cricopharyngeal myotomy for treatment of PES obstruction found that PESmax increased during swallowing of a 20-cc liquid bolus and pharyngeal constriction ratio (PCR) decreased, suggesting improved outcomes.

    ___X___ PCR has been shown to inversely covary with pharyngeal manometry pressure measures such that smaller constriction ratios were associated with higher manometry pressure measures during swallowing. In addition, normal PCR values were associated with normal manometry pressure values, whereas abnormal PCR values reflective of impaired pharyngeal constriction were associated with abnormally reduced manometry pressure values.

X Measures of PCR and pharyngeal area during referent hold position demonstrated that elderly individuals (>65 years) demonstrate significantly larger areas than younger individuals (≤65 years) and a greater distance between the hyoid and larynx during referent hold, suggesting that the pharynx is longer in elderly than in younger individuals as well.

33. c. does not allow us to expand interpretation to biomechanical deviations but can allow us to identify the presence or absence of aspiration.

34. a. the proportion of the total bolus entering the pharynx that was cleared during the swallow.

35. c. The maximum opening of the PES was greater than the normative measure values.

CHAPTER 9: OTHER TECHNOLOGIES IN DYSPHAGIA ASSESSMENT ANSWERS

1. esophagus

   1/3

   clavicle

   esophageal

2. a. can be used as a first-line tool to diagnose esophageal pathology in those with pill or solid food dysphagia complaints.

3. guided observation of swallowing

   Fiberoptic endoscopic evaluation of swallowing (FEES)

   oral

   pharyngeal

   esophageal

   esophageal

   esophagus

   esophageal

   gastric cardia

4. d. is a radiation-free option to the DSS for evaluation of some aspects of deglutition.

5. c. can be used to measure the quantity and location of a nuclear tracer, Tc-99mm, to identify aspiration.

6. __X__ Functional MRI enables investigation of neural pathways associated with deglutition activities.

   __X__ CT can be used to provide three-dimensional (3D) reconstruction of the aerodigestive tract anatomy and its function during swallowing.

   __X__ Dynamic MRI enables high-resolution study of the anatomic structures involved in deglutition.

7. a. velopharyngeal closure.

8. manometry

   36

   1

   5

   pharyngeal

sphincteric (UES)

esophageal

9. c. this method cannot be combined with manometry.

10. f. Responses (b) and (c) are correct.

11. e. All of the above responses are correct EXCEPT for (c).

12. FALSE

CHAPTER 10: THE TREATMENT PLAN: BEHAVIORAL APPROACHES ANSWERS

1. g. All of the above.

2. FALSE

3. c. an otolaryngologist.

4. f. Any of the above, depending on the patient.

5. TRUE

6. d. astrological.

7. a. a primary care physician.

8. FALSE

9. b. swallowing was shown to appear safer through the use of postural compensation methods.

10. e. can improve esophageal motility by providing electrical stimulation to the superficial musculature of the anterior neck.

11. f. Only (c) and (e) would be examples where behavioral management is considered inappropriate.

12. b. improve airway safety and swallow-related behaviors such as hyolaryngeal excursion during swallowing.

13. e. All of the above.

14. FALSE

15. FALSE

16. a. uniform and consistent use of the treatment protocol with all impaired individuals regardless of their diagnosis or current function level because these programs should work with everyone.

17. TRUE

18. a. flexible nasoendoscopy for direct imaging of pharyngeal structures.

19. d. high motivation to avoid long-term feeding tube use.

20. e. Responses (a) and (c) are both correct.

21. b. requires an intact lower motor unit to stimulate activation of the neuromuscular unit to enhance tone and strength in weakened muscles involved in swallowing.

22. e. Both (a) and (b) are correct.

23. FALSE

24. Functional electrical stimulation (FES) involves detecting the onset of a swallow using electromyography and impedance signals from the submental complex level to trigger a sequence of direct muscular stimulations to facilitate swallowing progress. In contrast, neuromuscular electrical stimulation (NMES) is an indirect form of muscle stimulation that can either be activated continuously or during swallow attempts using specific frequency-intensity-duration patterns. NMES is intended to enhance muscle contraction by increasing the number of motor action potentials generated by the muscles over which electrodes are placed.

25. __X__ Modify the size of bolus eaten (small bites versus large volume)

    __X__ Placing the bolus on the posterior left tongue, which appears stronger than the anterior tongue

    __X__ Modify bolus viscosity (liquid versus paste)

    __X__ Use of chemosensory stimulants such as sour or sweet

    __X__ Modify the temperature of the bolus (cold versus hot)

26. b. must consider the Newtonian characteristics of the bolus being modified.

27. __X__ Tilting the body laterally or posteriorly to divert the bolus away from the airway or toward musculature that appears intact and functional

    __X__ Anterior head flexion during each swallow to prevent aspiration before or during the swallow

    __X__ Providing jaw support to an infant for improved management of drinking through a nipple

    __X__ Rotating the head toward the side of impaired pharyngeal or laryngeal musculature to compress that side and encourage flow of the bolus through the functional or stronger side

28. __D__ This approach is used to increase displacement and duration of hyoid and laryngeal movement during the swallow to prolong PES opening. The patient is instructed to swallow and hold while the hyoid and larynx are raised and to relax after a prolonged duration after the swallow has completed (e.g., up to 1–5 s or so).

    __B__ Typically used with patients with airway closure timing delays or incomplete laryngeal closure during swallowing. The patient is instructed to put the bolus in the mouth and breath hold while swallowing and release the breath after the swallow is complete.

___E___ This method has been shown to be effective in patients with limited PES opening but with good control of oral structures such that they jut the jaw forward at the time of the swallow initiation.

___A___ Used typically in patients with weak pharyngeal constriction; patients are instructed to swallow as hard as they can and squeeze their swallow muscles harder.

___C___ Typically used with patients with airway closure timing issues or incomplete laryngeal closure during swallowing. The patient is instructed to bear down with great effort during swallowing to elicit supraglottic constriction for airway protection followed by an audible exhalation after the swallow is completed.

29. c. instructing the patient to swallow hard and squeeze her/his throat muscles.

30. ___X___ Reduce noise, light, and other distractions to enable orientation and focus on eating

___X___ Provide verbal cues (e.g., say his/her name, cue a behavior) or visual cues to the patient (hold up a card, gesture to the patient, etc.)

___X___ Stimulating the oral gums to provide mechanical stimulation to alert or orient oral structures during eating

___X___ Application of mechanical or vibratory stimulation to the faucial pillars to lower the mechanosensory threshold to stimulate onset of the swallow

___X___ Application of thermal stimulation via an icy laryngeal mirror to the anterior faucial pillars to improve swallow initiation

___X___ Transcranial magnetic stimulation to trigger pharyngeal constriction during swallowing

31. e. Both (a) and (b) are correct.

32. ___T___ It is important that members of the dysphagia team meet with and communicate the final treatment plan to the patient and her/his caregivers and respond to all related questions about the plan.

___T___ Pretreatment measures regarding the patient's swallowing quality of life and videofluoroscopic study can be compared with posttreatment studies and scores to determine progress or treatment outcome.

___F___ Differing opinions among team members regarding patient treatment methods or plans should not be documented.

___T___ The summary of findings for a patient with dysphagia should also include conclusions that the referring professional may not be able to independently determine, such as the etiology and severity of the impairment and its impact on nutrition and respiratory health and prognosis for improvement.

___F___ It is only important that the treatment plan be disseminated to the caregivers in the patient's immediate environment.

___T___ It may be important to post the treatment plan at the patient's bedside and include it in a hospital discharge plan.

   __T__   Recommendations for follow-up, if any, should be included in the report even though it is the responsibility of the patient's referring physician to monitor the patient and determine the need for follow-up visits or reevaluation.

   __F__   If a team sees a large number of patients, it is acceptable to allow time constraints to influence reduced priority of a thorough evaluation and critical review of each individual patient's situation in favor of improving efficiency.

33. TRUE

34. FALSE

35. TRUE

36. e. sending the patient to a different facility where her/his treatment will be carried out and evaluated posttreatment.

37. FALSE

CHAPTER 11: THE TREATMENT PLAN: MEDICAL AND SURGICAL ANSWERS

1. TRUE

2. a. benefit most from behavioral intervention using progressive lingual strengthening exercises or the Shaker exercises.

3. b. results in difficulty lubricating nonliquid boluses for effective swallowing clearance.

4. f. a patient exhibiting a cricopharyngeal bar and thinning of the posterior pharyngeal wall as well as an enlarged pharynx during quiet breathing.

5. c. characterized by cricopharyngeal hyperfunction.

6. TRUE

7. a. requires consistent daily use for 2 to 3 months for optimal management of reflux symptoms.

8. e. Only (a) and (b) are correct responses.

9. __X__ Proton-pump inhibitors (PPIs; e.g., omeprazole, pantoprazole, etc.)

   __X__ H2 blocker medications (e.g., famotidine, ranitidine, etc.)

   __X__ Endoscopic esophageal dilation

   __X__ Cricopharyngeal myotomy

10. e. prescription of pilocarpine medication.

11. FALSE (Schiedermayer et al., 2020)

12. g. All of the above are correct causes of achalasia.

13. c. cricopharyngeal muscle contraction.

14. __E__ Therabite jaw motion rehabilitation

    __C__ Cricopharyngeal myotomy

    __A__ Botox treatment administered to the orbicularis oris musculature

    __D__ Endoscopic balloon dilation

    __E__ Prosthetic palatal lift

    __B__ Velopharyngeal flap surgery

CHAPTER 12: AIRWAY CONSIDERATIONS IN DYSPHAGIA ANSWERS

1. __X__ Anterosuperior positioning of the hyolaryngeal complex under the base of tongue.

   __X__ Approximation of the true vocal folds, false vocal folds, and aryepiglottic folds

   __X__ Expiration preceding and following the swallow

2. __X__ Open heart surgery

   __X__ Diabetic coma

   __X__ Base-of-tongue cancer and surgery

   __X__ Loss of 10 lb during the past month

   __X__ Trach or ventilation tube in place

   __X__ Poor oral hygiene

   __X__ Chronic obstructive pulmonary disease

   __X__ Systemic inflammatory response syndrome

   __X__ Lung cancer

3. Auscultation is the method of listening to airway sounds using a stethoscope placed over the lateral larynx (cervical airway) or over the chest. Changes in the sound of laminar airflow during respiration, speaking, or swallowing can be used to determine whether sounds associated with aspiration can be detected. Placement of the stethoscope over the larynx or chest is used to listen for laminar versus nonlaminar airflow, but not for sounds associated with the swallow. Chest auscultation is also used to determine daily changes in respiratory patterns associated with aspiration and aspiration pneumonia. If sounds of aspiration or pneumonia are perceived, the patient may be recommended to undergo a chest radiograph.

4. __X__ Observe for struggle during eating, coughing, choking, and throat clearing

   __X__ Minimize distractions by maintaining a quiet environment and not talking during meals

   __X__ Do not leave the patient unattended or unobserved during meals

   __X__ Coordinate diet recommendations and restrictions with the physician's order for amount, frequency, and consistencies

   __X__ Oral care and hygiene before and after meals

   __X__ Position the patient at 90° in a chair, if possible, to maintain a safe upper body position

   __X__ Assess pulmonary status for clinical signs of aspiration

5. FALSE

6. Coughing

7. FALSE

8. FALSE

9. FALSE

10. TRUE

11. FALSE

12. FALSE

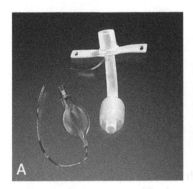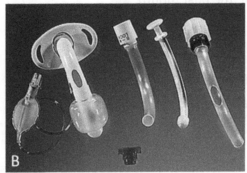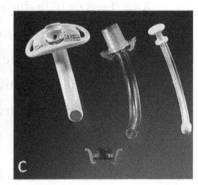

Figure 12–1

13. __A__ Cuffed tracheostomy tube

    __C__ Uncuffed/cuffless tracheostomy tube

    __B__ Fenestrated tracheostomy tube

14. a. **Cuffed tracheostomy tube:** Used to seal the airway and prevent aspiration of secretions into the lungs in an individual on positive pressure ventilation. These tubes are typically used in individuals in critical care settings or during surgical procedures requiring anesthesia. Patients are rarely sent home with a cuffed tube in place. A cuffed trach tube is typically deflated prior to eating.

    b. **Uncuffed/cuffless tracheostomy tube:** Used to maintain or provide an airway in an individual who is capable of breathing on his/her own but who requires secretion removal (suction) and airway maintenance. These tubes are typically used when an individual requires long-term airway support.

    c. **Fenestrated tracheostomy tube:** Used for weaning individuals from the tube and decannulation. These tubes may also be used so that an individual can more easily speak with a trach tube in place by allowing air to shunt through the larynx when the tracheostomy site is occluded. These tubes are typically left in place for only 3 to 5 days, as longer periods of time with capping the opening occur until the individual can tolerate breathing with the tube capped at the trach site for 18 to 24 hr.

15. – Habituation to the sensation of the trach tube within the trachea may lead to silent aspiration.

   – The trach tube may damage the respiratory mucosa lining the trachea, resulting in impaired mucociliary transport, important to moving particles and aspirated materials toward the larynx for expectoration.

   – The trach may tether the larynx, reducing hyolaryngeal excursion.

   – The presence of the trach tube may alter pharyngoesophageal pressure gradients important in transporting and clearing the bolus into the esophagus.

   – The presence of the trach tube may cause narrowing of the cervical esophagus.

CHAPTER 13: NUTRITIONAL CONSIDERATIONS IN DYSPHAGIA ANSWERS

1. FALSE

2. __X__ assess the patient's hydration needs.

   __X__ assess the patient's nutrition needs.

   __X__ translate restrictions recommended by the dysphagia specialists into a diet.

   __X__ contribute to transitions in dietary recommendations as needs change.

   __X__ consider ways to make the prescribed diet palatable and appealing to the patient.

   __X__ recommend modifications to tube feeding regimens for improved tolerance.

3. feeding

   anticipated

   amount

   nutrition

   hydration

4. d. All of the above.

5. __X__ Significant changes in a patient's weight trends and hydration

   __X__ Loss of more than 20% of an individual's usual weight

   __X__ Loss of 4 lb within 48 hr in a 100-lb person

   __X__ Rising blood urea nitrogen (BUN) level indicative of dehydration

6. TRUE

7. __C__ A positive acute phase protein that is used as an indicator of stress or inflammation

   __B__ Referred to as a "negative acute phase protein" that is considered to be a sensitive indicator of current protein status; it should never be considered alone as it can be lowered by inflammation, infection, or metabolic stressors regardless of nutritional status

   __D__ Elevated values occur in individuals suffering from dehydration in combination with other indications such as low urine output

   __A__ This measure reflects visceral protein status and can indicate nutritional risk when values are less than 3.2 to 3.5

8. FALSE

9. __X__ 6 oz servings of grains, emphasizing whole grains and higher fiber choices

   __X__ 2.5 cups of vegetables, emphasis on variety and color

   __X__ 2 cups from the fat-free or low-fat milk group that also includes fortified soymilk, cheese, yogurt, and tofu

   __X__ 5.5 oz equivalents from the meat and bean group (includes poultry, meats, eggs, and nuts)

   __X__ 5 teaspoons from vegetable oils

   __X__ 270 calories from discretionary calories including sweets, solid fats, and higher calorie foods

10. TRUE

11. FALSE

12. FALSE

13. d. recommending protein intake of 2.8 g/kg/day.

14. b. fluid needs increase as we age, in general.

15. FALSE

16. e. Both (a) and (b) are examples of noncommercial thickeners.

17. __B__ An individual who requires a relatively short duration of tube feeding can have a tube placed through the nose into the stomach through which feeds are administered into the stomach to bypass the upper airway.

   __D__ A feeding tube that is placed into the stomach through the mouth using one of two types of tubes, depending on whether the purpose is short term or long term.

   __C__ A long-term tube feeding option with the surgical placement of a tube into the stomach so that feeds can be administered directly into the stomach and the tube can be concealed when not in use.

   __A__ A patient who cannot take food through the digestive tract is provided her/his nutrition entirely through a large-flow-capacity vein.

CHAPTER 14: PEDIATRIC CLINICAL FEEDING ASSESSMENT ANSWERS

1. __X__ Sensory deprivation

   __X__ CNS disorders (e.g., cerebral palsy, brain malformations)

   __X__ Prematurity

   __X__ Genetic structural conditions (e.g., cleft palate, Pierre Robin)

   __X__ Social-behavioral maladaptation

   __X__ Cardiorespiratory compromise

   __X__ Gastrointestinal diseases (e.g., esophageal stenosis, GERD)

2. __X__ Malnutrition

   __X__ Dehydration

   __X__ Failure to thrive

   __X__ Respiratory complications

   __X__ Reduced quality of life for caregivers

3. d. one suck burst per second during nutritive sucking.

4. e. All of the response options are potential consequences.

5. Any of the following are correct responses:

   Sucking difficulties

   Gagging

   Unexplained food refusal

   Choking/coughing during meals

   Difficulties maintaining adequate caloric intake/weight (falls off the growth curve)

   Failure to thrive

   Recurrent pneumonias

   Lengthy or stressful mealtimes due to eating issues

   Drooling

   Reflux

   Vomiting

   High-risk medical diagnoses

   Frequent food regurgitation

6. FALSE

7. Any of the following are correct responses:

   Schedule for Oral–Motor Assessment (SOMA)

   The Pediatric Evaluation of Disability Inventory (PEDI)

   Oral–Motor/Feeding Rating Scale

   Multidisciplinary Feeding Profile

   Parental Feeding Questionnaire

   Dysphagia Disorders Survey (DDS)

   Pediatric Eating Assessment Tool (Pedi-EAT)

8. Physicians (developmental pediatrician, pediatric otolaryngologist, pediatric gastroenterologist, pediatric pulmonologist, pediatric neurologist, pediatric radiologist, pediatric psychiatrist)

   Nurse specialists

   Speech-language pathologist

   Occupational therapist with training and experience in feeding and dysphagia

   Behavioral psychologist/clinical psychologist

   Dietitian/nutritionist

   Social worker

9. perinatal

   neonatal

   hypoxia

   prematurity

   congenital

   illness

10. a. sensory processing disorders/hypersensitivity.

11. TRUE

12. FALSE

13. e. All of the responses above could be used to determine the nutritional status.

14. a. their weight-to-length ratio is <5% for age and gender (or body mass index once they turn 2 years of age).

    b. their weight is <5% for their gender and age.

    c. their weight percentage decreased by two or more standard deviations below the norm.

15. FALSE

16. TRUE

17. TRUE

18. parent

    nurse

    caregiver

    teacher

19. birth

    transitions

    foods

20. c. caregiver food preferences.

21. __X__ Types of foods eaten

    __X__ Amount of foods eaten

    __X__ Textures of foods eaten

    __X__ Physical environment of meals

    __X__ Family members present at meals

22. d. Eating Assessment Tool (EAT-10).

23. Any of the following are correct responses:

    A pale color of the skin may indicate iron-deficiency anemia

    Bruising may be due to vitamin K deficiency

    Bruising may also indicate physical abuse

    Skin rashes can be caused by deficiencies of essential fatty acids, zinc, or vitamins

    Skin and mucous membranes appear dry when inadequate fluid intake occurs (constipation may also occur)

    Children from developing countries may also show severe malnutrition with loose skin covering and decreased subcutaneous fat

    Excessive fluid retention causing edema due to poor protein intake (Kwashiorkor) or electrolyte imbalance

    Brittle, pale blond, and sparse hair is a sign of protein malnutrition

    Xerophthalmia, or dryness of the eyes, may be caused by vitamin A deficiency

    Conjunctivitis can result from malnutrition, affecting the immune system

24. __C__   The child exhibits a prolonged meal duration beyond 30 min.

   __B__   The child exhibits a rooting reflex upon gentle stroking of the cheek.

   __C__   The 8-month-old child exhibits aversion to rice cereal during a meal.

   __B__   The child exhibits a submucosal cleft upon inspection of the hard palate architecture.

   __A__   The child appears irritable and apathetic.

   __D__   The parent attempts to place additional food in the child's mouth while the child is still manipulating the last bolus in her/his oral cavity.

   __B__   The child exhibits oral hypersensitivity.

   __C__   The child exhibits successful finger feeding and cup drinking.

   __D__   The child continued to exhibit nutritional suck–swallow patterns at the time the parent thought the child was finished feeding.

   __A__   The child appears hungry and eager to eat.

   __A__   The child exhibits age-appropriate gross motor skills.

   __A__   The child's skin appears abnormally pale.

   __C__   The child shows a vertical jaw movement during chewing of food.

   __A__   The child appears anxious in the presence of food.

25. a. Phasic bite reflex—pressure on the gums causes rhythmic opening and closing of the jaws (gone by 9 to 12 months)

   b. Rooting reflex—a reflex present in newborns; when an infant's cheek is touched or stroked, he turns his head toward the touched side and begins to suck (3 to 6 months)

   c. Tongue protrusion reflex—forceful protrusion of the tongue, often in response to an oral stimulus (4 to 6 months)

   d. Suck/swallow reflex (4 to 6 months)

26. the types of foods that can be safely handled

27. __A__   Strong rooting reflex during gentle stroking of the cheek

   __C__   The primary central incisors may be present and lateral incisors erupting

   __A__   Tongue protrusion reflex in response to food other than liquid on the anterior tongue

   __B__   Tongue lateralization to manipulate food in the oral cavity is beginning

   __C__   Drinking from a cup independently

   __A__   Poor ability to sit upright independently

   __B__   Starting to open the mouth at the sight of food

   __C__   Develop a pincer grip on food (hold pieces between the thumb and index finger) during feeding

__B__ Stereotypical chewing (vertical jaw motion) and food manipulation are starting

__C__ Chewing patterns expand to lateral and possibly rotary movements

__B__ Increasingly able to sit independently and hold a bottle or cup

__A__ Bite reflex occurs in response to pressure on the anterior or lateral gums

__B__ Palmar grasp when picking up food

__A__ Insertion of the finger into the mouth triggers a sucking reflex

__C__ Primitive reflexes disappear

__A__ Anterior–posterior tongue mobility

__C__ Beginning to eat solid foods and biting off pieces to chew

__B__ Introduction of cereals begins

__A__ Oral hypersensitivity in response to foods other than liquids

28. d. 20 to 30 min.

29. a. Parent–Child Feeding Scale

30. TRUE

31. a. enables observation of the pharyngeal and esophageal phases of feeding.

32. c. choking/coughing.

33. FALSE

CHAPTER 15: ESOPHAGEAL PHASE DYSPHAGIA ANSWERS

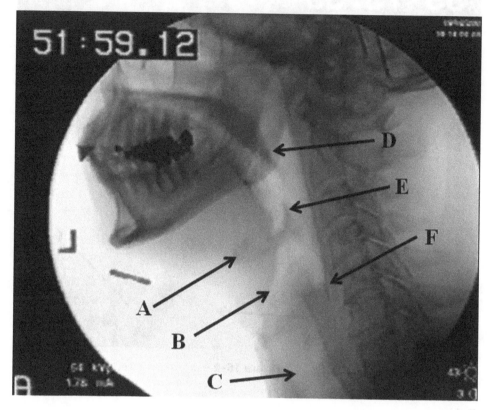

Figure 15-1

1. __C__ Trachea

   __D__ Soft palate

   __F__ Upper esophageal sphincter

   __B__ Larynx

   __A__ Hyoid bone

   __E__ Epiglottis

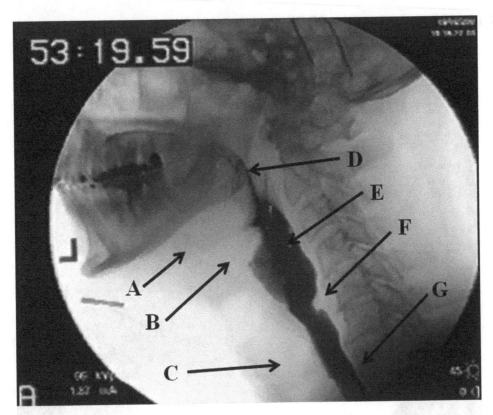

Figure 15-2

2. __E__   Bolus

  __G__   Esophagus

  __B__   Larynx

  __C__   Trachea

  __F__   Upper esophageal sphincter

  __D__   Oropharyngeal constriction

  __A__   Hyoid bone

3. a. upper esophageal sphincter and

    b. lower esophageal sphincter.

4. __X__   Food sticking in the throat

  __X__   Difficulty swallowing solid foods

  __X__   Food sticking at the level of the suprasternal notch

  __X__   Heartburn or indigestion associated with eating

  __X__   Sensation of a lump in the throat

5. gastroesophageal reflux disease (GERD)

   50

   edema

   esophageal body motility

   proton-pump inhibitor

6. FALSE

7. __X__ *Candida albicans*

   __X__ Chemoradiation therapy

   __X__ Food allergies

   __X__ Foreign body/pill impaction

8. esophagoscopy with biopsy.

9. c. oropharyngeal dysphagia.

10. a. inducing reflux.

    b. impairing esophageal motility and clearance.

    c. compromising the immune system predisposing to esophageal infection.

11. imposing caustic injury to esophageal tissues due to prolonged esophageal mucosal contact time.

12. a. taking pills in an upright position.

    b. taking pills with a large quantity of water (~120 cc).

    c. avoiding lying down for 30 min after taking pills.

    d. avoiding swallowing twice in a row causing deglutitive inhibition.

13. a. allergic rhinitis.

    b. eczema.

    c. asthma.

14. __X__ "Trachealized," or ringed, appearance to the esophagus during endoscopy

    __X__ Solid food dysphagia

    __X__ Esophageal strictures

    __X__ Esophageal food impactions

    __X__ Normal-appearing esophageal mucosa

15. gastroesophageal

    lower esophageal

    gastroesophageal

16. botulinum toxin (Botox)

    dilation

    squamous esophageal

    columnar gastric

    esophageal dilation

17. webs

    squamous

    proximal

    dilation

18. motility (IEM)

    manometry

19. __X__ Hypertensive LES

    __X__ Distal esophageal spasm (DES)

    __X__ Achalasia

    __X__ Nutcracker esophagus

20. ineffective esophageal motility (IEM)

21. a. **Esophagogastric junction outflow obstruction:** Characterized by an elevated median integrated relaxation pressure (IRP) in the primary and secondary position and ≥20% swallows with elevated intrabolus pressure in the supine position, with evidence of peristalsis. This occurs mostly in females later in life (59–69 years of age) without a known cause but potentially as a precursor to achalasia. Symptoms include dysphagia, chest pain, heartburn, and/or regurgitation.

    b **Nutcracker esophagus:** Esophageal contractions exhibit high-magnitude peristalsis greater than 180 mm Hg. Affected patients may complain of dysphagia and chest pain, and GERD may be diagnosed as well. The medication, sildenafil, has been associated with decreased peristaltic contraction amplitude, making it a treatment option.

    c. **Distal esophageal spasm:** Esophageal contractions are high amplitude AND nonperistaltic or simultaneous and sometimes give the appearance of a "corkscrew esophagus" when examined during an esophagram. Diagnosis is made using high-resolution manometry (HRM) with ≥20% premature contractions and distal contractile integral (DCI) of >450 mm Hg/s/cm^3. Patients complain of dysphagia and heartburn and may experience severe chest pain that rivals symptoms of a heart attack.

d. **Achalasia:** Characterized by degeneration of the myenteric plexus, resulting in impaired relaxation of the esophagogastric junction (EGJ) and the loss of organized peristalsis. Patients complain of a slow progression in onset of symptoms of dysphagia with solids and liquids without oropharyngeal transfer difficulties and may also complain of regurgitation, weight loss, chest pain, and heartburn.

22. b. Parkinson disease.

23. ___X___ Squamous cell carcinoma is a frequent tumor type associated with esophageal cancer.

   ___X___ Papillomas and cysts are examples of benign esophageal tumors.

   ___X___ Esophagoscopy is recommended for complaints of solid food dysphagia to rule out esophageal neoplasms.

24. esophagogastric junction (EGJ)

   peristalsis

   structural

   high-resolution manometry (HRM)

   barium esophagram (TBE)

25. d. Quantify the degree of opening and compliance of the lower esophageal sphincter (LES).

26. b. proximal esophagus spasm (PES).

CHAPTER 16: NEUROGENIC DYSPHAGIA ANSWERS

1. neurogenic, or neurological

2. 40

    80

    59

    91

    silent

    WITH

    CORRECTLY

    WITHOUT

    CORRECTLY

3. a. videofluoroscopy (dynamic swallow study).

    b. flexible endoscopic evaluation of swallowing.

4. 80

    15

    20

    aspiration pneumonia

    50

5. a. days.

6. __A__ Pharyngeal weakness

    __C__ Facial asymmetry and weakness

    __E__ Silent aspiration

    __B__ Tongue asymmetry and fasciculations

    __D__ Tongue deviation away from the side of cortical damage with normal symmetry and tone of the tongue

    __B__ Difficulty forming a cohesive bolus

    __A__ Weak cough

7. __X__ Difficulty initiating a swallow

    __X__ Prolonged pharyngeal transit

    __X__ Tongue pumping (several posterior tongue movements prior to triggering a swallow)

    __X__ Delayed airway protection relative to bolus transit

8. upper

lower

fasciculations

atrophy

aspiration

9. ___X___ Evidence of primitive reflexes (tongue pumping, sucking, tongue extrusion)

___X___ Impaired coordination of oropharyngeal movements

___X___ Respiratory function requiring a tracheostomy or ventilator

___X___ Delayed onset of swallowing

___X___ Injury to cortical and subcortical structures

10. plaques

conduction

WORSENS

11. solid

liquid

12. spasticity

13. ___X___ Abnormal posture

___X___ Impaired oral stage function

___X___ Laryngeal penetration/aspiration

___X___ Impaired mastication

14. pneumonia

feed oneself

15. medications

xerostomia

pills

13

barium tablet

16. inflammatory myopathies caused by autoimmune conditions

inflammatory cells, such as B and T cells, infiltrate skeletal muscle

17. diverticulum

18. Duchenne muscular dystrophy (DMD)

    dystrophin

19. cricopharyngeal

    dilatation

    pseudodiverticula

20. pharynx

    upper esophageal sphincter (UES)

    50

21. antibodies against the muscle membrane of the neuromuscular junction causing inadequate production of acetylcholine (the neurotransmitter released from neurons into the neuromuscular junction that stimulates muscle contraction)

    progressive fatigue or muscle weakening with prolonged duration of neuromuscular activation

    positioning

    dietary modifications

22. __B__ The most common of the muscular dystrophies, which does not occur until adulthood. It is associated with progressive muscle wasting and weakness with impact on swallowing affecting the pharynx and upper esophageal sphincter most.

    __C__ This disease is caused by a genetic defect for the protein in muscles called dystrophin, resulting in rapid worsening of the disease. It affects boys rather than girls due to the pattern of inheritance such that girls are carriers only. Onset is usually prior to the age of 6 years.

    __A__ This disease is inherited and typically does not occur until middle age with onset of eyelid drooping (ptosis) initially followed by onset of swallowing difficulties related to pharyngeal weakening.

CHAPTER 17: DYSPHAGIA IN HEAD AND NECK CANCER PATIENTS ANSWERS

1. FALSE

2. TRUE

3. PRE-

4. 23

   44

   71

5. a. Tumor location

   b. Tumor size (the larger the tumor, the more severe the dysphagia)

6. FALSE

7. a. Surgery

   b. Chemotherapy

   c. Radiation

   d. Chemoradiation

8. a. hyolaryngeal elevation during the swallow.

   b. tongue stabilization during eating.

9. a. Impaired or absent hyolaryngeal elevation during the swallow

   b. Impaired ability or inability to open the pharyngoesophageal sphincter

   c. Impaired tongue mobility

   d. Impaired bolus preparation and propulsion

   e. Pharyngeal residue

   f. Aspiration after the swallow

   g. Impaired tongue sensation, including general sensation and taste

10. __X__ Odynophagia

    __X__ Mucositis

    __X__ Anorexia

    __X__ Xerostomia

    __X__ Infections in the oral and pharyngeal cavities

11. a. Microstomia (small lip opening) impairing introduction of a bolus into the mouth

    b. Reduced or impaired sensation to the lip(s)

    c. Difficulty keeping food in the oral cavity

    d. Reduced intra-oral pressure generation for bolus propulsion into the pharynx

12. __X__ Odynophagia

    __X__ Nasal regurgitation

    __X__ Reduced or absent hyolaryngeal excursion

    __X__ Impaired tongue mobility

    __X__ Loss of smell

    __X__ Impaired pharyngeal constriction

    __X__ Xerostomia

    __X__ Pseudoepiglottis

    __X__ Posterior pharyngeal wall tethering during swallowing

    __X__ Oronasal fistula and nasal residue

13. __X__ Mucositis

    __X__ Odynophagia

    __X__ Reduced or absent general sensation

    __X__ Reduced or absent hyolaryngeal excursion

    __X__ Impaired tongue mobility

    __X__ Pharyngeal residue

    __X__ Impaired pharyngeal constriction

    __X__ Silent aspiration

    __X__ Fibrosis of soft tissues

    __X__ Pharyngoesophageal stenosis

14. a. decrease weight loss.

    b. maintain nutritional needs.

    c. maintain hydration levels.

15. __E__ Removal of the mandible

    __C__ Only the laryngeal structures invested with cancer are removed and reconstruction of the remaining tissues involved in voice production, typically requiring a permanent tracheostomy due to inadequate airway opening

__B__ Removal of cancer involving the superior portion of the larynx such as the ventricular and aryepiglottic folds, epiglottis, and hyoid bone

__D__ Removal of a tumor near the jugular foramen involving the CNs IX and X or in the infratemporal fossa

__A__ Removal of the entire larynx and reconstruction of its attachments within the pharynx, including creation of a permanent tracheostomy to separate the airway from the esophagus

16. TRUE

17. 8 to 12 weeks

tissue fibrosis of deglutition musculature

18. to preserve tissues and organs to improve functional outcomes rather than remove tissues resulting in impaired function.

FREQUENT

INCREASED

19. a. Base-of-tongue dysfunction

b. Reduced pharyngeal constriction

c. Reduced laryngeal excursion

20. DECREASE

tumor site

pharyngeal

aspiration

silent aspiration

cough response

INCONSISTENT

21. __B__ This method is used to recruit as many motor units as possible during swallowing in those with weakened oropharyngeal musculature, particularly those with difficulty swallowing their secretions or with excess saliva production.

__A__ This method is used to enhance recruitment of pharyngeal constrictor muscle activation during swallowing by reducing participation of the base of tongue in oropharyngeal constriction during swallowing.

__C__ This method is used to improve reduced superior and anterior excursion of the hyolaryngeal complex associated with piriform sinus residue.

22. a. **PHYSICIAN GOAL:** to eradicate the cancer and save the patient's life while consideration is given to minimizing functional impairment that will result from medical and surgical treatment approaches

    b. **SPEECH-LANGUAGE PATHOLOGIST GOAL:** to optimize eating function in the face of remaining structural and physiologic deficits from treatment of the head and neck cancer

23. a. maintenance of nutritional needs.

    b. maintenance of hydration needs.

CHAPTER 18: LARYNGOPHARYNGEAL REFLUX ANSWERS

1. the flow of stomach contents backward through the esophagus into the laryngopharynx.

2. __X__ Dysphonia

   __X__ Laryngeal granulomas

   __X__ Subglottic stenosis

3. three

4. __A__ Heartburn

   __A__ Esophagitis

   __B__ Daytime reflux

   __A__ Nighttime reflux

   __A__ Reflux occurs in supine position

   __B__ Reflux occurs in upright position

   __A__ Prolonged episodes of reflux

   __B__ Brief episodes of reflux

   __A__ Body mass index increases prevalence

   __B__ Body mass index does not increase prevalence

   __A__ Lower esophageal sphincter dysfunction is an etiology

   __B__ Esophageal dysmotility is not an etiology

   __B__ Upper esophageal sphincter dysfunction is an etiology

5. FALSE

6. __X__ Hoarseness or a problem with your voice

   __X__ Clearing your throat

   __X__ Difficulty swallowing food, liquid, or pills

   __X__ Troublesome or annoying cough

   __X__ Sensations of something sticking in your throat or a lump in your throat

7. __X__ vocal fold edema

   __X__ granuloma/granulation

   __X__ ventricular obliteration

   __X__ pseudosulcus (infraglottic edema)

   __X__   erythema/hyperemia

   __X__   diffuse laryngeal edema

   __X__   thick endolaryngeal mucus

   __X__   posterior commissure hypertrophy

8. a. **Pseudosulcus:** A furrow is observed along the medial vocal fold edge extending along both the membranous and cartilaginous portions. This is in contrast to sulcus vergeture, which exhibits a furrow along the medial membranous portion of the vocal fold only. Pseudosulcus is a sign most often associated with LPR.

   b. **Reinke's space edema:** Swelling of the vocal folds due to excessive production of a gelatinous material within the superficial lamina layer of the lamina propria in the vocal folds. This space between the middle and deep layers that comprise the vocal ligament and the epithelial layer is referred to as Reinke's space. The swelling and thicker substance within this layer add mass and stiffness to the vocal folds so that the frequency of vibration is lowered, resulting in a lower pitched voice that is sometimes rough in quality due to asymmetries in vibration. This finding is a sign of laryngeal tissue irritation from smoking and from exposure to stomach contents.

   c. **Vocal fold granuloma:** These are benign mass lesions that develop as an inflammatory response to chronic irritation or mucosal injury. They most often occur in the posterior larynx over the vocal process where they make contact during voice production. Their name comes from the granulated appearance of the mucosal tissue surface. The most common causes are from endotracheal trauma; chronic excessive vocal fold overclosure in the posterior larynx during talking, coughing, or throat clearing; and from LPR.

9. 24-hr dual-probe pH testing

   ABOVE

   IS NOT

   ABOVE

   manometry

   DOES NOT

   mucosal airway

   5

10. adenocarcinoma

11.   __X__   Avoid alcoholic beverages

      __X__   Avoid lying down less than 3 hr after eating

      __X__   Avoid acidic foods such as citrus and tomatoes

      __X__   Stop smoking

      __X__   Bring weight to normal standards

    __X__   Elevate the head of the bed by 6 in.

    __X__   Avoid wearing tight clothing

12. TRUE

13. proton-pump inhibitor medications

    TWICE

    16

    2

    6

    30

    45

14. Nissen fundoplication

    hiatal hernia repair

CHAPTER 19: SPINAL ABNORMALITIES IN DYSPHAGIA ANSWERS

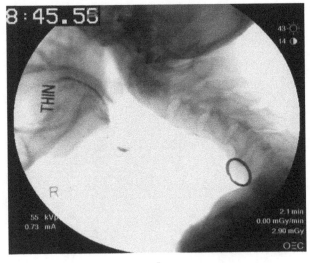

A

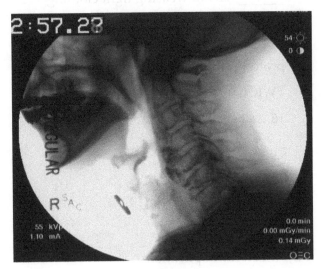

B

1. CONVEX

   KYPHOSIS

   OSTEOPHYTES

2. 27

   86

   C5/C6

3. __X__ Narrowing of the pharyngeal diameter

   __X__ Bolus obstruction in the UES or esophagus

   __X__ Impeded epiglottic inversion

4. TRUE

5. e. All of the above responses.

6. b. progressively form within the pharyngeal mucosa and submucosa.

7. c. pharyngeal transit time, hyoid elevation

8. 47

   21

   zero

9. __X__ Neurodegenerative disease

__X__ Cerebrovascular accident

__X__ Cricopharyngeus muscle dysfunction

__X__ GERD

10. FALSE

11. __D__ Reduced UES opening during the swallow

__C__ Reduced base of tongue motion

__B__ Reduced pharyngeal muscle function

__F__ Solid food dysphagia with narrowed pharynx due to obstructive pathology

__E__ Poor epiglottis deflection

__A__ Delayed swallow onset, or reduced sensation to bolus residue

12. osteophytectomy

epiglottectomy

enteral

References

Belafsky, P. C., Postma, G. N., & Koufman, J. A. (2002). Validity and reliability of the Reflux Symptom Index (RSI). *Journal of Voice, 16*, 274–277.

Feng, F. Y., Hyungjin, M. K., Lyden, T. H., Haxer, M. J., Worden, F. P., Feng, M., . . . Eisbruch, A. (2010). Intensity-modulated chemoradiotherapy aiming to reduce dysphagia in patients with oropharyngeal cancer: Clinical and functional results. *Journal of Clinical Oncology, 28*, 2732–2738.

Koufman, J. A. (1991). The otolaryngologic manifestations of gastroesophageal reflux disease (GERD): A clinical investigation of 225 patients using ambulatory 24-hour pH monitoring and an experimental investigation of the role of acid and pepsin in the development of laryngeal injury. *Laryngoscope, 101*(Suppl. 53), 1–78.

Langerman, A., MacCracken, E., Kasza, K., Haraf, D. J., Vokes, E. E., & Stenson, K. M. (2007). Aspiration in chemoradiated patient with head and neck cancer. *Archives of Otolaryngology–Head and Neck Surgery, 133*, 1289–1295.

Langmore S. E., McCulloch, T. M., Krisciunas, G. P., Lazarus, C. L., VanDaele D. J., Pauloski, B. R., & Doros, G. (2016). Efficacy of electrical stimulation and exercise for dysphagia in patients with head and neck cancer: A randomized clinical trial. *Head and Neck, 38*(Suppl. 1), E1221–E1231.

Leonard, R., & Belafsky, P. (2011). Dysphagia following cervical spine surgery with anterior instrumentation: Evidence from fluoroscopic swallow studies. *Spine, 36*(25), 2217–2223. https://doi.org/10.1097/BRS.0b013e318205a1a7.

Logemann, J. (1983). *Evaluation and treatment of swallowing disorders*. College-Hill Press.

Sapienza, C., & Wheeler, K. (2006). Respiratory muscle strength training: Functional outcomes versus plasticity. *Seminars in Speech and Language, 27*, 236–244.

Schiedermayer, B., Kendall, K. A., Stevens, M., Ou, Z., Presson, A. P., & Barkmeier-Kraemer, J. M. (2020). Prevalence, incidence, and characteristics of dysphagia in those with unilateral vocal fold paralysis. *Laryngoscope, 130*(10), 2397–2404. https://doi.org/10.1002/lary.28401

Smith-Hammond, C. A., New, K. C., Pietrobon, R., Curtis, D. J., Scharver, C. H., & Turner, D. A. (2004). Prospective analysis of incidence and risk factors of dysphagia in spine surgery patients: Comparison of anterior cervical, posterior cervical, and lumbar procedures. *Spine, 29*(13), 1441–1446.

Teraguchi, M., Yoshimura, N., Hashizume, H., Muraki, S., Yamada, H., Minamide, A., . . . Yoshida, M. (2014). Prevalence and distribution of intervertebral disc degeneration over the entire spine in a population-based cohort: The Wakayama Spine Study. *Osteoarthritis and Cartilage, 22*(1), 104–110.

U.S. Department of Health and Human Services and U.S. Department of Agriculture. (2015). *2015–2020 Dietary guidelines for Americans, 8th edition*. https://health.gov/our-work/food-nutrition/previous-dietary-guidelines/2015

Willaert, A., Jorissen, M., & Goeleven, A. (2015). Swallowing dysfunction in myotonic dystrophy: A retrospective study of symptomatology and radiographic findings. *Acta Oto-Rhino-Laryngologica Belgica, 11*, 249–256.